Practical Oral Medicine

Quintessentials of Dental Practice – 10
Oral Surgery and Oral Medicine – 3

Practical Oral Medicine

By
Iain Macleod
Alexander Crighton

Editor-in-Chief: Nairn H F Wilson
Editor Oral Surgery and Oral Medicine: John G Meechan

Quintessence Publishing Co. Ltd.

London, Berlin, Chicago, Paris, Milan, Barcelona, Istanbul,
São Paulo, Tokyo, New Delhi, Moscow, Prague, Warsaw

British Library Cataloguing-in Publication Data

Macleod, Iain, Dr
  Practical oral medicine. - (Quintessentials of dental practice ; 10.
  Oral surgery and oral medicine ; 3)
  1. Oral medicine
  I. Title II. Crighton, Alexander III. Wilson, Nairn H. F. IV. Meechan, J. G.
  617.5´22

ISBN 1850970653

Copyright © 2006 Quintessence Publishing Co. Ltd., London

ISBN 1-85097-065-3

Foreword

The everyday clinical practice of dentistry includes aspects of oral medicine. Lesions and abnormalities of the soft tissues of the mouth and orofacial region are common, with many conditions being indicative of systemic disease and disorders. Knowledge, understanding and the effective practice of oral medicine are therefore integral to the provision of holistic oral healthcare.

Oral medicine, in common with all other aspects of dentistry, continues to evolve at an ever increasing rate. This volume of the unique *Quintessentials of Dental Practice* series captures the essence of modern oral medicine for, in particular, the busy practitioner. From immunological problems through lumps and bumps, infections and white patches to premalignant lesions and oral cancers, together with sections on oral pigmentation, disorders of salivary glands and salivation, facial pain, neurological disorders and complementary therapies, this *Quintessentials* volume provides essential chairside information and guidance. Aficionados of Quintessence books and, in particular, the *Quintessentials* series will be pleased to recognise all the qualities they have come to expect: succinct, easy to digest, up-to-date text, well illustrated with high quality graphics and images.

This book is both a valuable, close-to-hand reference text and a pleasure to indulge in over the one or two evenings it takes to complete the cover to cover read. A gem of a book in the world-class *Quintessentials* series. I hope you enjoy and discover new dimensions to oral medicine from this excellent addition to the ongoing series.

Nairn Wilson
Editor-in-Chief

Acknowledgements

To Enid and Emilia, without whose support over the years this work would not have been possible.

Contents

Chapter 1
Introduction and Oral Medicine in Clinical Practice

Aim

The aim of this chapter is to outline the development of oral medicine and to describe the oral medicine consultation.

Outcome

After reading this chapter you should understand the importance and structure of an oral medicine consultation.

Introduction

Oral medicine has been defined as 'the speciality of dentistry concerned with the health care of patients with acute or chronic, recurrent and medically related disorders of the oral and maxillofacial region, and with their diagnosis and medical management. It is also concerned with the investigation, aetiology and pathogenesis of these disorders leading to understanding that may be translated into clinical practice. Oral medicine is a clinical and academic speciality that is dedicated to the investigation, diagnosis, management and research into medically related oral diseases, and the oral and facial manifestations of systemic diseases. These include diseases of the gastrointestinal, dermatological, rheumatological and haematological systems, autoimmune and immunodeficiency disorders, and the oral manifestations of neurological and psychiatric diseases.'

The practice of oral medicine requires a sound knowledge of medical science in order to provide a rational approach to diagnosis and clinical management. It is also essential for the competent provision of dental care to those with special needs - patients with physical, mental or medical disability.

Oral medicine permeates virtually all branches of dentistry and many areas of medicine. It can be regarded as the interface between medicine and dentistry. This book covers in a practical manner the scope of oral medicine most likely to be encountered in a dental setting. It does not pretend to be all-inclusive, and readers are advised to make reference to more specialist publications where appropriate. Some of these are suggested at the end of each chapter. In addition, some conditions more usually managed by maxillofacial, ear, nose and throat (ENT) or plastic surgery have been deliberately excluded.

The Oral Medicine Consultation

The initial appointment is often the most important time in patient's management. This meeting sets the tone for all remaining visits. The patient forms opinions about the expertise and competence of the practitioner. The clinician forms views about the patient and his or her problem. As communication, empathy and trust form a large part of treatment, it is important that the process gets off to a good start on both sides.

An effective practitioner will manage to put patients at their ease. This can establish trust, allowing full disclosure of information relevant to the problem to be obtained. Many factors are important in this. The following can all play a part:
- body language
- seating position and arrangement
- dress
- language.

One of the most important lessons for the inexperienced clinician to learn is when not to talk and to encourage the patient to keep providing information. It is important to retain control of the consultation, however, and not be afraid to redirect patients when they digress from pertinent information.

The stages of the consultation are as follows:
- greeting
- introduction
- information-gathering
- review and discussion
- conclusion and future planning.

Each stage is important and will take place at every consultation, but the emphasis on each will vary between initial and review consultations.

Greeting

This is the first contact between the patient and the clinician. It may occur when collecting the patient from the waiting area or as the patient enters the surgery. The clinician should greet the patient in an open and welcoming manner, introducing himself and all other people present at the consultation by giving their name, position and their role. The patient should be seated comfortably, facing the clinician in preparation for the next stage of the consultation. If the patient has brought a supporter, ideally he or she should be seated able to face and communicate with the patient and the clinician. Where possible all individuals in the consultation room should be easily visible to the patient, as this helps relaxation.

Introduction

The clinician should outline the purpose of the appointment - for example, a referral from another practitioner, a review of investigation results or treatment progress. An outline of the process of the consultation is appropriate at the initial visit, informing the patient of the different stages to expect – history, review and the possible need for discussion with other health care workers, special investigations and arrangements for management. Many complaints from patients relate to communication failures rather than to treatment problems. It is important that the patient and the clinician are equally clear about the purpose and scope of the consultation at this visit.

Information-Gathering

The history should follow a standard format to enable reproducibility. A sample history-taking plan is given in Table 1-1. Some aspects of the history process will be identical for all patients and some - in particular, the history of the presenting complaint - will vary according to the problem. Some of the key issues in a patient with recurrent oral ulceration will be of little relevance in someone with chronic facial pain, but a thorough medical and social history will be important for both. In this book, where there is information required for a particular oral complaint, the specific history points to cover will be reviewed in the appropriate chapter. All sources of information including, if appropriate, the opinions of the supporter, can be important and should be canvassed. At the end of the history, it is helpful to read back to the patient the clinician's understanding of the presenting problem, its course and management to this point. Any misunderstandings or misinterpretations on the part of the clinician can then be set aside at an early stage.

A full clinical examination of the head and neck should then take place. Depending on the differential diagnosis, the expertise of the clinician, local

Table 1-1 **Information to be obtained from each patient**

For each patient the following information must be obtained

- Name, age and gender

- Presenting complaint (PC) *or* reason for referral (RR) if symptom-free

- History of presenting complaint (HPC)
  - Who noticed the lesion/condition? – when it was noticed
  - Site of problems – intra-oral/extra-oral
  - Symptomatic – what symptoms reported? Duration of symptoms?
  - Periodicity of symptoms – variations during the day/day to day/week to week?
  - Precipitating and relieving factors – foods/eating, analgesia effect? Others?
  - Treatments tried so far – success? the most helpful? unhelpful?
  - For painful lesions – score/10 – At worst? At best? Today? Average? *(10/10 – worst pain imaginable, 0/10 – no pain)*
  - Associated symptoms – for example, skin, muscle/joint, genital, gastrointestinal system

- Past medical history
  - Serious illnesses and operations in the past
  - Current attendance at hospital, clinic or GP – why?
  - Current medications – (no dosage needed)
    NB: Record generic drug name only, not drug 'trade' name
  - Allergies to medicines – record the effect the drug produced as well

- Systems enquiry: *Check particularly:*
  - Cardiovascular   Angina, previous myocardial infarction
  - Respiratory   Asthma/chronic obstructive pulmonary disease (use of inhalers?), smoker (what quantity?)
  - Gastrointestinal   Dyspepsia, ulcers, altered bowel habit, bleed PR
  - Urinary   Prostatism (men!)
  - Skin   Rashes, itch, eczema
  - Specific diseases   Rheumatic fever, jaundice, diabetes, epilepsy
  - Family history   illnesses known in blood relatives? (myocardial infarction, cerebrovascular accident, diabetes)
  - Social history   Who is at home? Are they well? Actual/desired employment? Happy at work? Alcohol consumption history

Examination, Diagnosis and Treatment

- Clinical findings on examination
    - Observation of the patient – appearance, demeanour
    - Extra-oral findings – nodes, salivary swellings, tenderness of soft tissues, cranial nerve function, pigmentation changes, scars
    - Intra-oral findings – full mucosal examination, general dental condition, periodontal and dental charting as needed
    - Results of special investigations today for example, salivary flow, Schirmer test, cranial nerve exam

- Further investigations ordered - imaging, histopathology and biopsy

- Treatment plan
    - Note if discussed with colleague
    - Bullet point or number items
    - Record those completed today
    - Outline purpose of next visit

- Sign and date record in case record

- Ensure appropriate letters are dictated

clinical practice and facilities, a more complete physical examination of the patient may also be appropriate (Figs 1-1 to 1-3).

Review and Discussion

After the examination it is useful to summarise the key points elicited in the examination and relate these to the history. From this the patient can see how the clinician has reached the offered diagnosis, or where there is a need for proposed investigations. In most oral medicine problems, the patient will be the 'key worker' in the delivery of treatment. It is therefore essential that the patient accepts the diagnosis and treatment plan suggested. In addition, the patient should understand the likely outcome, effects and timescale of the proposed treatment. The patient and, if appropriate, the supporter should be invited to ask questions about the diagnosis and proposed treatment.

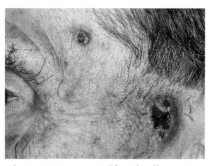

Fig 1-1 Two typical basal cell carcinomas on the left temple area – such a finding can occur during the routine inspection of the face. By permission of Oxford University Press from "Oral Pathology 4/e" edited by Soames, JV & Southam, JC (2005).

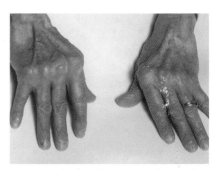

Fig 1-2 The hands can reveal a number of physical signs and are easy to examine in the otherwise dressed patient. In this case they show the typical joint changes and deformity of rheumatoid arthritis.

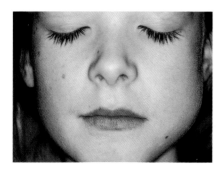

Fig 1-3 Chronic swelling of a buccal lymph node – in most cases this arises in response to dento-facial infection but can also be a manifestation of malignancy, such as lymphoma or, in this case, rhabdomyosarcoma.

Where possible, written information should be given. This may be a full information leaflet, if available, but simply writing the name of the diagnosis and proposed treatment on paper to hand to patients can be helpful. This will aid understanding of their condition and ultimately their involvement in and compliance with treatment.

Conclusion and Future Planning

At the end of the initial consultation the patient should be made aware of investigations planned, the likely duration of the treatment and the planned intervals for review. It is useful to explain why a particular interval is chosen – for example, two-month intervals rather than one month - as this will help the patient understand the treatment process. Similarly it is important to ensure that the patient knows how to contact the clinician should the situation or condition change so that a new review interval or unscheduled appointment can be arranged. If it is decided to refer to a more appropriate specialist, the reason and mechanism for this should be clearly explained. The general medical practitioner can often play a pivotal role in the provision of care for oral medicine conditions, in many cases providing the treatment for the patient according to the treatment plan. If urgent medication is required, it may be necessary to contact the general medical practitioner asking for a particular treatment to be made available quickly or to dispense directly to the patient from the clinic.

At the end of the consultation patients should have a clear understanding of their future care plan. Notes should be completed promptly and letters sent to appropriate people, usually including the general medical practitioner. The general medical practitioner is often the only person aware of the 'bigger picture' in the patient's care and, as a consequence, should routinely be included in all correspondence.

onclusions

· Communication skills are an essential part of oral medicine.
· A full history, including a medical and social history are necessary for all patients.
• All health-care practitioners should be kept updated with changes in the patient's care plan.

Further Reading

Schouten BC, Eijkman MA, Hoogstraten J. Dentists' and patients' communicative behaviour and their satisfaction with the dental encounter. Community Dental Health 2003;20:1,11–15.

Piasecki M. Clinical Communication Handbook. London: Blackwell Scientific Publications, 2003 (ISBN 0632046465).

Chapter 2
Immunological Problems of the Oral Mucosa

Aim

The aim of this chapter is to review immunological oral disease, including lichen planus, oro-facial allergic disorders, recurrent aphthous stomatitis, mucocutaneous autoimmune disorders, vasculitis and systemic autoimmune disorders presenting in the head and neck region.

Outcome

After reading this chapter you should be able to understand the features of immunological disease affecting the head and neck, together with the systemic effects of these diseases and factors influencing their presentation or management.

Introduction

Immunological oral disease is a very broad subject. Many mucosal and periodontal problems are caused either directly or indirectly by the host's immune system. Some oral manifestations represent mouth changes as part of a whole body process, and other conditions produce lesions or symptoms mainly or only in the mouth. In this chapter immunological problems, including the oral effects of allergy, will be reviewed together with the oral mucosal effects of immunological reactions to the oral mucosa.

Orofacial Allergic Disorders

Allergy is usually classified by its four main methods of presentation:
- type 1 - immediate (anaphylactic)
- type 2 - autoimmunity
- type 3 - immune complex disease
- type 4 - delayed hypersensitivity.

Many patients presenting with allergy-related disease will have a history of atopy, such as eczema or asthma. The presentation of allergy in the oral soft tissues may be very varied. Gingival hyperplasia may be found in patients with allergic nasopharyngeal reaction, resulting in tissue desiccation secondary to mouth-breathing. Gingival erythema may be the result of a toothpaste allergy, often leading to a significant plasma cell infiltrate and the clinical appearance of a desquamative gingivitis. Allergy can be the basis of many other oral mucosal diseases not primarily considered 'allergic' disorders. These include recurrent aphthous ulceration and lichen planus. There is also an association with geographic tongue, but there is no good evidence suggesting a causal relationship.

Type 1 Reactions

These are produced by the rapid movement of fluid into the tissues from the circulation and are characterised by rapidly increasing swelling of the tissues and, following removal of the stimulus, gradual resolution over a period of hours. In this condition the transudation of fluid into the tissues from the capillaries is more rapid than the capacity of the lymphatics to drain the fluid away. This can be seen in patients with angio-oedema of the lips or tongue such as may be triggered by ACE-inhibiting drugs or C_1 esterase dysfunction.

Angio-oedema

In this condition the patient will report rapid lip swelling over less than an hour with gradual resolution over the remainder of the day. Most patients with these symptoms do not seem to have a recognisable trigger, and empirical management with a long-acting, non-sedating antihistamine is the mainstay of treatment.

The combination of angio-oedema with bronchospasm, vasodilatation and rapid hypotension suggests another type 1 reaction – anaphylaxis. This reaction may follow dental treatment, such as a reaction to latex containing gloves worn by the dental team, or more rarely a local anaesthetic injection. Environmental triggers, such as a bee or wasp sting, are also possibilities, and an anaphylactic reaction should never be discounted only because no drug has been administered to the patient.

Type 2 Reactions

There are no oral conditions commonly associated with a type 2 reaction.

Type 3 Reactions

In the oral tissues the type 3 reaction is uncommon. This involves an antibody combining with an antigen in the circulation and the resulting immune complex becoming deposited in the blood vessel walls. This activates the complement cascade locally, causing perivascular inflammation of the tissues. In the mouth the most frequent clinical picture seen is the widespread inflammation and ulceration associated with erythema multiforme.

Erythema Multiforme (Fig 2-1 and Fig 2-2)

Patients with this condition present to many different medical specialties, depending on the most involved tissue. Dermatologists see those patients presenting only with skin lesions, ENT surgeons manage patients with nasopharyngeal involvement and urologists deal with lesions limited to the genitals. When all of the above sites are involved the condition is termed 'Stevens-Johnson syndrome'. In the mouth the patient classically presents with a haemorrhagic pseudomembrane on the lips, together with oral ulceration not dissimilar to that seen in a primary herpetic gingivostomatitis. Erythema multiforme is usually self limiting within 10-14 days. Patients are best managed with supportive treatment, including fluids and analgesia. There is now good evidence

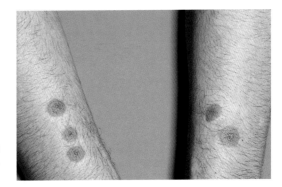

Fig 2-1 'Target' lesions on the arms of a patient with erythema multiforme.

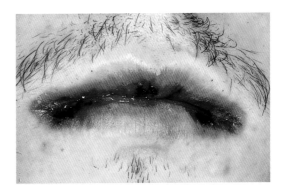

Fig 2-2 Erythema multiforme presenting with ulceration and crusting of lips.

that many of the patients with oral symptoms have the episode triggered by herpes simplex virus, and patients with recurrent episodes of erythema multiforme in the mouth often benefit from low-dose, prophylactic aciclovir for six months. Mycoplasma pneumonia is a less commonly seen trigger, and drug reactions are unusual. Occasionally symptoms are severe enough to warrant a reducing course of a systemic steroid – for instance, prednisolone combined with an antiviral drug such as aciclovir or famciclovir. In other patients the erythema multiforme may result from an environmental trigger, and formal allergy testing can be considered for patients not helped by aciclovir prophylaxis.

Type 4 Reactions

These are sometimes known as contact allergy or delayed hypersensitivity and present on the skin with itch, erythema and vesiculation. Whereas the latter two are found in oral reactions, itch is uncommon except when the lips or perioral skin are affected. There are many possible triggers for type 4 reactions, and in dentistry these include:
- metals
- dental materials
- latex
- food allergies.

Metal Allergies (Fig 2-3)
Nickel and palladium are the metals most commonly implicated in oral allergic reactions. Palladium is present in bonding alloys used in restorative procedures. Nickel is a constituent of most metal alloys and is thus found in stainless steel dental instruments, orthodontic appliances and cobalt chromium dentures. Contact sensitivity to nickel is reported in up to 15% of the population. After visiting the dentist the nickel sensitive patient may experience perioral discomfort, angular cheilitis and lip erythema, which may be mistaken for a recurrent herpetic lesion. The use of latex-free rubber dam on a plastic frame can reduce contact between the dental instruments and the perioral tissues, consequently reducing post-treatment symptoms.

Dental Materials
Many dental materials contain organic and synthetic elements implicated in sensitivity reactions elsewhere in the body. Inside the mouth reactions are unusual, although hypersensitivity to eugenol, acrylic monomer and composite resins, such as 2-hydroxyethyl methacrylate, have all been reported. Chemicals used in dental procedures, such as formaldehyde and sodium hypochlorite, have also been shown to sensitise some staff and patients.

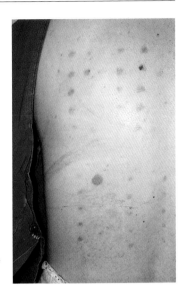

Fig 2-3 Patch-testing: this shows a positive result (round patch of erythema) as a result of mercury sensitivity from amalgam.

Lichenoid reactions to amalgam and, less commonly, to composite restorative resins are discussed more fully later in the section on white lesions (Chapter 5). Typically the reaction to the material will resolve on its removal, but this can be a slow process taking up to six months for complete resolution.

Latex (Fig 2-4)

Many of the perioral features seen in type 4 reactions to latex gloves are identical to those described above for nickel-sensitive patients. Barrier methods, such as the non-latex dam, are useful here as well, but for the latex-sensitive patient the dental team involved in delivering clinical care should use latex-

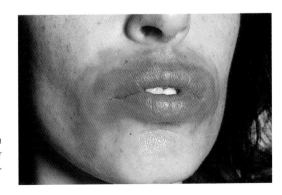

Fig 2-4 Perioral dermatitis in patient with a latex sensitivity after being treated by a dentist wearing rubber gloves.

free gloves, such as the nitrile variety. Vinyl gloves are not now recommended, as they are not guaranteed to be impervious to body fluids and thus do not offer a satisfactory level of staff protection. Patients who are latex-sensitive must also be protected from other latex-containing materials in dentistry. These include local anaesthetics where latex is used in the cartridge seals, prophylaxis cups and orthodontic elastics. The use of gutta percha remains controversial in this patient group.

Food Allergies

Food allergies have been blamed for many medical problems. A small proportion of patients have a true sensitivity to food constituents or additives, but many more claim this problem. For a true allergy to exist, not only must the suspected reaction resolve on withdrawal of the putative agent, but it must also recur on re-exposure. Coeliac disease is a true food allergy to the alpha gliaden component of wheat. There are a few oral diseases associated with allergies to food components. The most notable of these is orofacial granulomatosis (OFG) where, in some study populations, a significant proportion of patients show immediate or delayed reactions on testing to common food preservatives and flavourings. Preservatives such as benzoic acid (benzoates) and sorbic acid (sorbates) are common culprits, together with other additives in the E210-219 series. Flavouring agents, such as cinnamon and chocolate, and a variety of other everyday environmental items, such as balsam of Peru and colophony, can be identified as environmental triggers in OFG patients. Dietary and environmental agent exclusion are often the best management path for patients with this problem, but this can be difficult in view of the ubiquitous nature of the allergens in contemporary living. Food allergies are also worth considering in some patients with recurrent aphthous stomatitis and angiooedema, particularly in those who respond poorly to conventional treatment.

Fixed Drug Eruptions

These are not commonly found in the oral environment, but more recently the potassium channel blocker nicorandil has been associated with tongue ulceration. The ulcer is usually shallow, about 1cm in diameter, on the lateral margin of the tongue, exceedingly painful and poorly responsive to conventional therapies. As most patients have been taking the drug for some time before symptoms develop many physicians fail to associate the ulceration with the drug. Stopping the nicorandil produces a rapid improvement in symptoms and rapid healing of the ulcer. Re-introduction of the drug is quickly followed by the return of the ulcer on the same site. If a drug reaction for an oral lesion is suspected, the dental practitioner must always discuss the problem with the patient's physician to ensure that a suitable alternative therapy is arranged for the continuing medical problem, usually angina.

Orofacial Granulomatosis (Figs 2-5 to 2-7)

Orofacial granulomatosis is a chronic granulomatous condition limited to the face and mouth. It presents with a prolonged oedematous swelling of the lips and perioral soft tissues. Most often there is an associated angular cheilitis, with exfoliative lip dermatitis, fissuring and perioral erythema seen in a few cases. Typical intra-oral findings include mucosal oedema leading to a 'cobblestone' pattern together with mucosal tags and aphthous-type oral ulceration. In a minority a marked gingival erythema is noted. Rarely fistulae can develop from the mouth into the pharynx or, more distressingly, the facial skin.

The oral lesions are due to giant cell granulomas located within the lymphatic channels draining the affected tissue. These act as a 'plug', preventing normal transudated tissue fluid passing back to the circulation through the lymphatics. There does not seem to be an increase in fluid entering the tissues, and the swelling seen is due to its gradual accumulation over time.

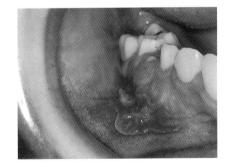

Fig 2-5 Tissue tags on the buccal sulcus in a young patient with orofacial granulomatosis OFG)

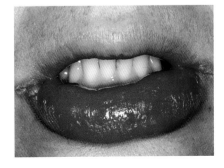

Fig 2-6 Chronic swelling of lower lip with associated bilateral angular cheilitis. These appearances are suggestive of orofacial granulomatosis (OFG) or oral Crohn's disease. This feature is also known as cheilitis granulomatosa.

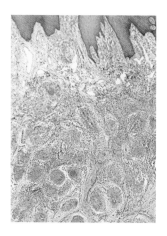

Fig 2-7 H&E stained section through the tongue demonstrating granulomatous inflammation from a patient with orofacial granulomatosis (OFG). A similar appearance would be seen in Crohn's disease, and this specimen demonstrates how the granulomata lie fairly deep within the tissue and, as a consequence, the need for a large biopsy to allow diagnosis.

Consequently any effective treatment must prevent granuloma formation and thus allow the gradual reopening of the lymphatics. For this reason changes in appearance following any intervention can take many weeks to produce a clinical improvement. The condition can appear at any age, but most patients are in the first three decades of life. Biopsy does not always demonstrate the classical giant cell granulomas unless it is performed deep into the most affected tissue area, often as far as the muscle layer. However, distended lymphatics are usually seen. Similar pathological findings can be present in sarcoidoisis, and this condition must always be included in the differential diagnosis of chronic facial swelling. Much confusion exists within dentistry in differentiating OFG from Crohn's disease. The label 'oral Crohn's' is given when oral lesions are found in association with similar findings on biopsy, endoscopic or radiological changes noted in the 'hidden' gastrointestinal tract. Crohn's disease, like OFG, is not a condition with a single cause and is likely to represent a group of conditions producing similar clinical findings. As with OFG, suggested causes for Crohn's disease include food allergies, an infectious agent (possibly an atypical mycobacterium) or an idiosyncratic reaction to measles vaccine. Investigations for OFG patients should include a dietary history, especially carbonated beverage intake, note of any gastrointestinal symptoms of altered bowel habit or rectal bleeding, unusual breathlessness and skin lesions. Laboratory investigations vary widely between clinicians, but the serum angiotensin-converting enzyme (ACE) is an important marker for sarcoidosis in many patients and is essential for every OFG patient. It is also important to check ferritin, red-cell folate and vitamin B_{12} levels, as low levels of these may suggest occult gastrointestinal tract disease. Additionally, low ferritin levels will exacerbate any angular cheilitis or oral ulceration present and iron must be replaced as part of the patient's overall management. An important investigation is allergy testing to identify a suitable exclusion regimen where possible. In many patients the trigger is never found, and treatment is limited to reducing the cosmetic and psychological problems caused by the lip swelling. The use of repeated intralesional injections of a potent steroid such as triamcinolone can gradually produce an improvement in the patient's appearance, although the benefit is usually lost over a few months. The condition seems to fade with time in many patients. However, if the swelling has been present for many years the chronic inflammatory changes will result in fibrin and possibly collagen deposition in the tissues. This makes the disfigurement permanent. In these cases the best cosmetic outcome is achieved through surgical filleting of the lip tissue.

Summary

- Allergy is probably under-recognised as a cause of oral disease and symptoms.
- Patch-testing is of limited value in identifying triggers for allergic problems.
- Dietary and environmental exclusion trials are often the most useful way to identify certain disease triggers.

Lichen Planus (Figs 2-8 to 2-12)

This is a relatively common mucocutaneous condition affecting between 2-4% of the population. It can present as a purely skin problem, mucosal problem or a combination of both. Many patients present complaining of recurrent oral ulceration, and lichen planus should, therefore, be included in the differential diagnosis for this symptom. The skin lesions usually comprise an itchy, violaceous, macular-papular rash most frequently affecting the flexor surfaces of wrists, shins and midriff regions. However, other sites may be affected – such as the nails, which become dystrophic, or the scalp, leading to hair loss (alopecia). In approximately half of the patients presenting with dermatological manifestations of lichen planus the oral mucosa will also be affected. Only 10-30% of those presenting with oral lichen planus develop cutaneous manifestations, however, and this may reflect a different trigger for the two presentations.

The oral presentation of lichen planus is most often with white patches and striae, affecting any site, but typically in a symmetrical and bilateral distri-

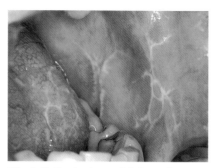

Fig 2-8 Reticular oral lichen planus.

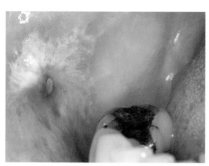

Fig 2-9 Lichenoid reaction on buccal mucosa due to amalgam sensitivity. Note the close proximity of the large amalgam restoration adjact to this lesion.

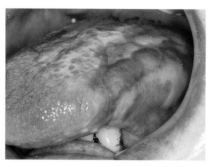

Fig 2-10 Major erosive oral lichen planus.

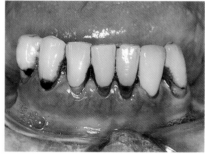

Fig 2-11 Desquamative gingivitis in a patient with oral lichen planus. A similar appearance may also be seen in patients with mucous membrane pemphigoid and can also occur as a result of a local hypersensitivity reaction. By permission of Oxford University Press from "Oral Pathology 4/e" edited by Soames, JV & Southam, JC (2005).

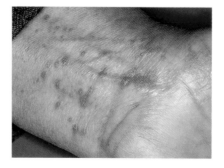

Fig 2-12 Typical purplish macular-papular rash on the flexor surface of wrist in cutaneous lichen planus.

Table 2-1 **Lichen planus subtypes**

- Reticular
- Plaque
- Papular
- Atrophic
- Erosive
- Bullous

bution. The appearance can vary. At least six forms have been described (Table 2-1). A clear division into these types is often difficult, and examination may reveal more than one variant in a patient. Furthermore, classification by type has little influence on clinical management apart from erosive lesions, which may carry a 1-2% risk of malignant transformation.

Although the diagnosis of lichen planus is often made on clinical grounds alone, a biopsy should be undertaken routinely to assess any underlying dysplastic change. Once the diagnosis has been confirmed, treatment depends on symptoms (see appendices A and B). Generally, there is a slightly higher incidence of oral lichen planus in females than males, but unlike the cutaneous disease, which usually resolves after a few months, the oral lesions can persist for many years.

Lichenoid Reactions

These are so named because of their similarity, both clinically and histologically, to lichen planus. The difference is that a lichenoid reaction is associated with some provoking agent. One way in which to consider the issue is that lichen planus is a lichenoid reaction in a patient where the trigger has not yet been identified. A lichenoid change represents a type 4 hypersensitivity reaction. A variety of drugs, foodstuffs and dental materials, in particular amalgam, have been implicated in the development of these types of lesions.

The differentiation of a lichenoid reaction from lichen planus can be difficult and may seem arbitrary, although an association between the appearance of the lesion and the start of a certain medication may be suggestive. Any contact between affected areas and large, often old, amalgam restorations should also raise suspicion. The replacement of these restorations with a different material usually produces a speedy resolution, confirming the cause and providing the treatment. Patch-testing of patients with suspected lichenoid reactions is time-consuming but may help to track down possible sensitisers in an otherwise intractable condition.

Graft-Versus-Host Disease

Graft-versus-host disease (GVHD) can present with oral and cutaneous lichenoid appearances as part of a graft-versus-host reaction in patients who have received an allograft bone-marrow transplant, especially from peripheral blood stem-cell transplants. GVHD oral lesions can be managed in a similar fashion to oral lichen planus, but in most cases the oral effects are mild when compared to the systemic consequences of this disease. The physicians will use potent systemic immunosuppressive drugs to control GVHD. If an oral lesion proves resistant, intralesional steroids may have a useful role.

Recurrent Oral Ulceration (ROU)

Recurrent oral ulceration is not synonymous with recurrent aphthous stomatitis – this is only one form of recurrent oral ulceration. Patients with intermittent lesions frequently attend when no ulceration exists, and the history is very important in planning investigations and therapy. Where a conclusion is difficult to reach it is better to review the patient at the next appearance of the lesion so that clinical and possibly pathological findings can be added to the information from the history.

Many conditions produce oral ulceration that may present on more than one occasion, and these are summarised in Table 2-2.

Non-Aphthous Ulceration

Traumatic Ulceration

This is a very common clinical presentation with repeated ulceration from an ill-fitting denture, sharp tooth or appliance being mistaken for an aphthous pattern. However, any persisting ulcer must be considered carefully. If the mucosa is not obviously healing within two weeks of removing the suspected source of trauma then an incisional biopsy of the lesion is indicated to exclude malignant disease. In some patients the mucosal trauma may be deliberate (factitious ulceration) when an individual has discovered a perceived gain from having an oral lesion. This may be a child getting time away from school to attend the clinic or may represent a reaction to significant psychological stress, such as bullying or abuse. In both adults and children the help of an experienced clinical psychologist is invaluable in the assessment and management of the patient and their problems.

Table 2-2 **Recurrent oral ulceration**

- Non-aphthous
  - Traumatic ulceration
  - Lichen planus
  - Vesiculobullous disorders
  - Viral infections

- Aphthous stomatitis (RAS)
  - Major aphthae
  - Minor aphthae
  - Herpetiform aphthae
  - Behcet's syndrome
  - Reiter's syndrome

An important variation of traumatic ulceration is the traumatically induced aphthous ulcer. Here the patient has a tendency to produce aphthous type ulceration, but this is only expressed when the mucosa is injured, for example by parafunctional clenching. The mild mucosal trauma then results in aphthae forming along the occlusal line of the lips and buccal mucosa together with the lateral margin and tip of the tongue. This clinical pattern strongly suggests traumatically induced aphthae and is best managed with a lower soft-bite splint possibly combined with a tricyclic drug such as amitriptyline at night.

Other Mucosal Disease

Mucosal conditions other than aphthae can produce recurrent oral ulceration. For this reason it is important to elicit the ulceration pattern in the history. As an example, vesiculobullous lesions will produce recurrent oral ulcers on sites often associated with aphthae. However, most patients will be aware that the ulcer is preceded by a blister, which bursts to produce the ulcer. It is important to make this distinction, and every patient presenting with a history of recurrent oral ulceration should be asked whether a blister formed before the ulceration. The most common mucosal disease producing a history of recurrent oral ulceration is lichen planus. Here the ulceration is usually in the same place each time and occurs in sites typical of lichen, such as the buccal mucosa or lateral margins of the tongue.

Recurrent Aphthous Stomatitis (Fig 2-13 to Fig 2-15)

Aphthous oral ulceration can be subdivided into two main groups, major and minor. Major aphthous ulcers are the less common variety but cause much distress. These painful ulcers are characterised by their size and dura-

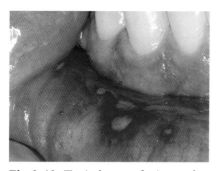

Fig 2-13 Typical crop of minor aphthous ulcers affecting the lower labial mucosa.

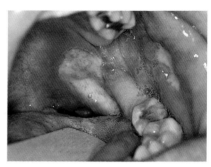

Fig 2-14 Major aphthous ulceration of the soft palate and anterior fauces. Such lesions may mimic an oral malignancy and can result in fairly significant tissue loss and tend to heal with scarring.

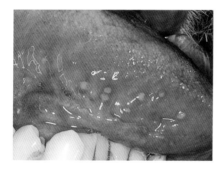

Fig 2-15 Herptiform aphthous ulceration affecting the ventral surface of the tongue.

tion, often persisting for several weeks before healing, often with residual scarring. Typically the ulcers are a centimetre or greater in diameter and can occur on any part of the oral mucosa. Usually they prove resistant to common topical treatments. Minor aphthous ulcers are round, painful shallow ulcers on the non-keratinised oral mucosa that typically last for 10-14 days. After a variable ulcer-free period the ulcers return and the cycle repeats many times, but no scarring of the mucosa is seen. On some occasions, the ulcer pattern is described as herpetiform, where many small ulcers appear on the oral mucosa, often coalescing to form one large ulcerative area. In the initial stages the many small ulcers are said to resemble a herpetic gingivostomatitis, but there is no known role for herpes simplex virus in this condition.

The cause of aphthous ulceration is not known, but it appears that the Langerhans cells in the epithelium are triggered to activate CD4 and CD8 lymphocytes against a specific area of the mucosa. This results in epithelial cell death and consequent ulceration. Although HLA associations vary widely between races, there appears to be a genetic component to this condition, with most sufferers having one or both parents with a history of similar problems. This genetic tendency is modified by systemic and local factors in the host to produce the clinical picture at presentation. If patients report severe oral ulceration for most of their life it is likely that the genetic factors predominate in the trigger for their ulcer formation. Where the pattern of ulceration has changed, however, a systemic or environmental factor may be responsible for the change, acting to amplify the genetic predisposition. Consequently it may be possible to modify and improve the clinical pattern of ulceration and quality of life. Most patients find the occasional mouth ulcer no more than a nuisance, but the longer the ulcer duration and the shorter the ulcer-free period, the more likely they are to seek help. The degree of disability experienced by some patients with near-continuous oral ulceration should not be underestimated.

Aphthous-type ulceration is not limited to the mouth and can often be described in the pharynx by patients and is seen throughout the colon at endoscopy. Some individuals are affected from early childhood, but most children presenting to clinics are between eight and 12 years old. Commonly this is shortly before the start of a period of rapid skeletal growth. During this time body iron stores fall and this seems to be associated with enhanced mucosal vulnerability and an increased frequency of ulceration. Iron deficiency (not anaemia) is a common finding in many patients whose pattern of oral ulceration has changed. The reason for the iron deficiency changes with gender and age but should always be explored. Menstrual blood loss is the most common explanation in younger women. Young male patients and many older patients of both sexes may, however, present with iron deficiency from upper gastrointestinal bleeding, most commonly gastric erosions or peptic ulcer disease. The use of NSAID medication for treatment of arthritis makes this a common finding in the elderly. In this group, it is important to identify lower gastrointestinal bleeding, as this is often associated with premalignant colonic polyps or colonic cancer. Thus, a change in the ulcer pattern in older patients can be very significant.

Other systemic disease can also be responsible for alterations in oral ulceration pattern. Gastrointestinal problems, including malabsorbtion, such as coeliac disease, may also influence the course of ulceration. Oral ulceration is also found in ulcerative colitis, often when the colitis itself is problematic. The role of hormonal changes is less clear, particularly the influence of the menstrual cycle. Some patients clearly have pre- or perimenstrual ulceration over many months. The response to endocrine manipulation in these individuals though is rarely encouraging, but usually get significant remission during pregnancy. Smoking cessation is another trigger for the onset of significant aphthae in a cohort of patients, with some citing this as the sole reason for reacquiring the habit. Finally, allergy testing has a role in identifying patients where food additives or other environmental agents, such as nickel, may be promoting the ulceration.

Management of Aphthous Ulcers

It is important to have a strategy for the investigation and management of patients with aphthous ulceration. The aim of treatment should not necessarily be to render the patient ulcer-free but to achieve an adequate quality of life. This balance can only be judged by the patient. The possibility of an underlying medical problem or deficiency state must be explored and managed. After this, the key principles of treatment are to use the least potent treatment consistent with adequate ulcer control. This suggests that topical steroids must be preferred to systemic treatment. Many preparations are available, but high-potency steroids, such as betamethasone, clobetasol and triamcinolone, are preferred. Other topical treatments, such as tetracycline or ciclosporin mouth washes, are rarely used now, as effective patient compliance with the required regimens is poor. However, chlorhexidine mouthwash can be beneficial in some cases. Where significant symptoms persist, systemic treatment should be considered. Such treatment should be started only after a full discussion with the patient as to the short- and long-term consequences of immunosuppressive therapy. Often a trial of systemic therapy, such as prednisolone with azathioprine, for a period of three to six months allows an assessment of the benefit of this treatment. The effects on the patient's quality of life can then be judged before considering longer-term use. In some patients with prolonged major aphthae, such as those with Bechet's or Reiter's syndromes (Table 2-3), substantial benefit can be derived from other immune-modulating drugs, including colchicine, thalidomide and dapsone.

Summary

- Recurrent aphthous stomatitis is only one form of recurrent oral ulceration.
- Aphthae are probably genetically determined but facilitated by local environmental changes – for example. trauma, iron deficiency, coeliac disease.
- Always exclude systemic disease when investigating aphthae.

Table 2-3

Bechet's syndrome
- Oral Ulceration (major, herpetiform)
- Genital ulceration (often painless)
- Uveitis (posterior)
- Young adult (20-30's)
- Male 3:1 female
- Associated with HLA B5 & Bw51

Reiter's syndrome
- Oral ulceration painless and superficial
- Conjunctivitis, urethritis and arthritis
- Link to infections suggested
  - mycoplasma
  - gonococcal disease
- Associated HLA B27

- The lowest-potency treatment compatible with a good quality of life for the patient should be used – for instance, topical rather than systemic steroid treatment.

Vesiculobullous Disorders (Fig 2-16 to 2-21)

Vesiculobullous disorders are characterised by rapidly developing, fluid-filled swellings of the skin or mucous membranes that burst to leave an area of ulcerated tissue. Patients can be referred suffering from recurrent oral ulceration. For this reason it is important to ask all patients presenting with recurrent oral ulceration as to whether they have blisters that burst to form ulcers. There are many causes of blistering lesions of the oral mucosa, and these are summarised in Table 2-4. The more common forms presenting in the mouth are:
- angina bullosa haemorrhagica
- mucous membrane pemphigoid
- pemphigus vulgaris.

Direct immunofluorescence can be used to differentiate sub-epithelial blistering from intraepithelial disease by staining IgG, IgM, IgA or C_3 antibody bound to the tissue. Unfortunately this produces broadly similar findings for many of the subepithelial conditions. This can make understanding of the

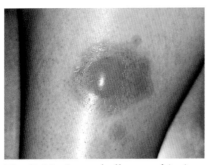

Fig 2-16 Intact bullae on shin in a patient with bullous pemphigoid.

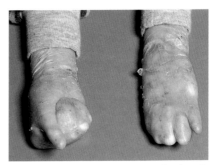

Fig 2-17 Severe scarring to the hands in a young girl affected with epidermolysis bullosa. By permission of Oxford University Press from "Oral Pathology 4/e" edited by Soames, JV & Southam, JC (2005).

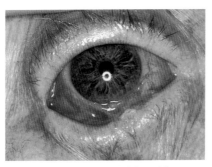

Fig 2-18 Conjunctivitis with some scarring in a patient with mucous membrane pemphigoid.

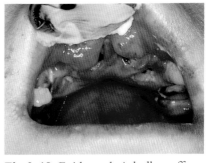

Fig 2-19 Epidermolysis bullosa affecting the oral tissues. Note the simple action of elevating the lip can cause trauma to the tissues and result in severe scarring.

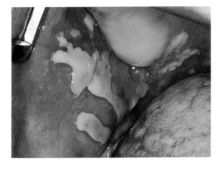

Fig 2-20 Irregular ulceration of the buccal and palatal mucosa covered in a thick fibrinous slough in patient with pemphigus.

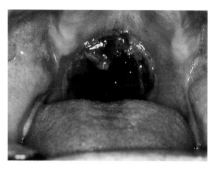

Fig 2-21 Large blood filled blister on the soft palate, which in this case represents angina bullosa haemorrhagica. A similar appearance can occur in thrombocytopenia or mucous membrane pemphigoid.

Table 2-4 **Vesiculobullous lesion of the oral mucosa (common lesions in bold type)**

Intraepithelial

Pemphigus - Vulgaris
          - foliaceus
          - vegetans
          - Familial benign

Darier's disease

Subepithelial

Pemphigoid - Mucous membrane
          - bullous

Angina bullosa haemorrhagica
Dermatitis herpetiformis
Linear Ig A disease
Epidermolysis bullosa
Bullous lichen planus

clinical presentations, course and sequelae of the different disorders difficult. In fact the antigens targeted by the autoantibodies in the vesiculobullous lesions are directed at different and highly specific epitopes on transmembrane proteins, such as laminin 5 and desmoglein, in the intercellular region. An apparently small change in the epitope position involved can make the difference between a relatively benign or an aggressive disease course, tissue-scarring or uneventful healing. Some of the vesiculobullous disorders do not form true visible bullae, although these are seen histologically.

Angina Bullosa Haemorrhagica

This is the most commonly encountered bullous condition in dental practice with subepithelial blisters similar in nature to pemphigoid. They have no characteristic immunofluorescence staining and are not associated with any blistering skin condition. Many patients are aware of the recurrent formation of blood–filled blisters a few millimeters in diameter from time to time. These are commonly on the buccal mucosa, but larger lesions can present on the soft palate, particularly in the older patient. These are reported to be triggered by eating and the bullae are short-lived, with most rupturing within the hour, giving the patient a taste of blood in their mouth. Medical therapy seems to have little to offer the patients with angina bullosa haemorrhagica, so reassurance is usually the only treatment required.

Mucous Membrane Pemphigoid

Pemphigoid describes a range of conditions characterised by loss of adhesion between the epithelium and the connective tissue along the line of the basement membrane. The blisters formed in subepithelial conditions contain either colourless or bloodstained (red) fluid. The blisters are also relatively robust and may persist for several days before rupturing, leaving ulcers that take several weeks to heal. These ulcers are similar to aphthae in their symptomatology. Pemphigoid occurs when an autoantibody, usually IgG but potentially IgM or IgA, is targeted at a 230kda protein component in the hemidesmosome in the mucosal basement membrane.

Depending on the epitope targeted in the basement membrane, mucous membrane pemphigoid can present either with or without scarring on healing. Pemphigoid can be associated with similar blistering and scarring on mucous membranes other than the oral soft tissues. Of importance is conjunctival disease with scar formation (synechia) between the mucosal surfaces, which eventually leads to corneal opacity. An ophthalmological opinion should be sought for all patients presenting with oral pemphigoid lesions. Cutaneous pemphigoid (bullous pemphigoid) involves a 180 kda antigen and can produce oral lesions, but these are not present in every case. A wide range of antigens can be targeted in pemphigoid, and the spectrum of clinical presentations varies with the epitope involved.

Pemphigus Vulgaris

Pemphigus is the least common of the major vesiculobullous lesions to affect the mouth and usually presents intra-orally with a white area of oral mucosa. This is easily lost, leaving an area of erosion or ulceration. The white colour-change is the result of fluid accumulation within the epithelium, obscuring the vascular connective tissue beneath. Pemphigus vulgaris is unusual among oral bullous disorders in that it often presents first in the oral mucosa before skin and other mucosal lesions appear. Any intra-oral soft tissue site can be involved, including the attached gingivae, presenting as a desquamative gingivitis. In pemphigus an IgG autoantibody targets desmoglein 3 in the desmosomes between epithelial cells, resulting in loss of cell adhesion. This allows mucosal erosions to form with minor trauma. Skin lesions develop subsequently in many patients and the condition is eventually lethal, due to a combination of cutaneous blistering and fluid loss, infection and toxicity to the drug therapy. In a small number of patients the onset of pemphigus is associated with occult malignant disease (paraneoplastic pemphigus). This should always be considered when making a diagnosis of pemphigus and particularly when there is an unusually aggressive clinical course.

Other Vesiculobullous Disorders

Linear IgA disease (LAD), dermatitis herpetiformis (DH) and bullous lichen planus (BLP) are less common conditions presenting with intra-oral blister formation. All present with sub-epithelial blistering and seem to involve the 180 kda bullous pemphigoid antigen as part of their epitope profile. On direct immunofluorescence IgA is the autoantibody detected in LAD and DH. Whereas the pattern of antibody distribution is contiguous along the basement membrane in LAD it is deposited in a granular pattern in DH. Dermatitis herpetiformis is strongly associated with coeliac disease, and as a consequence there is often a useful improvement in symptoms when the patient rigidly adheres to a gluten-free diet. Linear IgA disease, however, can be very troublesome to manage, often necessitating a combination of immunosuppressant drugs to achieve a useful clinical improvement. Bullous lichen planus is an unusual variant of lichen planus where the characteristic histopathological picture is combined with a clinical history of bullae formation in the lichenoid area. No autoantibody is detected on direct immunofluorescence.

Management of Vesiculobullous Lesions

When bullae are present it is good practice to take a quality clinical photograph to illustrate the lesion in case the diagnosis is later subject to review. A biopsy of either an intact bulla or perilesional tissue is essential. Both routine histopathology and direct immunofluorescence should be requested. Remember that biopsies of ruptured bullae are of little help, as the epithelium is often missing. Where possible, further investigation into the epitope targeted can give information useful in determining the likely clinical course. It is always important to liaise with other health care workers appropriate to the patient's symptoms and condition. This may be a dermatologist where pemphigus or linear IgA disease is found, a gastroenterologist in dermatitis herpetiformis and an ophthalmologist in mucous membrane pemphigoid. To control the oral lesions, whether true bullae or a desquamative gingivitis pattern, a graded approach to the use of steroids and other immunosuppressive drugs is recommended. Appendix B details a common approach to steroid therapy for oral medicine problems, and the dose of steroid and nonsteroidal immunosuppressive drugs are titrated to achieve the desired clinical effect.

Summary

- Vesiculobullous disorders may be referred as recurrent oral ulceration.
- An intact bulla or perilesional tissue for direct immunofluorescence, as well as standard histopathology, is needed to make a diagnosis.
- Oral bullae may precede skin lesions in some patients, especially those with pemphigus.
- Close liaison with a dermatologist and ophthalmologist may be required for some patients with vesiculobullous disorders.

Systemic Autoimmune Conditions

Patients with systemic autoimmune disease often have oral, salivary or facial changes associated with their condition (Table 2-5). In Sjögren's syndrome, for example, these may be the most troublesome aspects of the disease. Systemic autoimmune conditions of interest include:
- lupus and connective tissue diseases
- organ-specific autoimmune diseases
- vasculitic diseases.

Table 2-5 **Head and neck features in systemic autoimmune conditions**

Rheumatoid Arthritis	direct disease effects - TMJ arthritis - associated connective tissue disease (Sjögren's) - amyloidosis indirect disease effects - drug effects - ulcers, lichenoid reactions - poor care delivery - attendance - reduced oral care - reduced host defences (including candida, caries)
Sjögren's	dry mouth dry eyes swallowing and taste disturbance salivary gland swelling salivary gland lymphoma
Systemic lupus erythematosis	oral or facial lupus lesions butterfly rash on face 'lichenoid' lesions of the mucosa
Scleroderma	limitation of access to the mouth widened PDL space on radiograph

Lupus and Associated Syndromes (Figs 2-22 and 2-23)

This includes rheumatoid arthritis (RA), systemic and discoid lupus erythematosis (SLE/DLE), Sjögren's syndrome (SS), scleroderma and mixed connective tissue disease (MCTD). These are all multisystem disorders and are best thought of as a spectrum of disease, with each 'syndrome' having features most prominent in one tissue or body system. SLE is the most 'general' and discoid lupus the most localised. As an example, dry mouth and salivary involvement can occur in any of these conditions, but they are mainly associated with and most common in Sjögren's syndrome. Each condition is linked with one or more autoantibodies. These are listed in Table 2-6. It

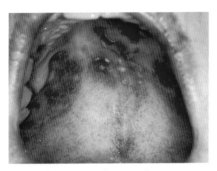

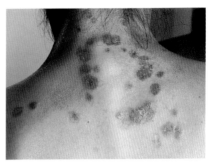

Fig 2-22 Extensive erosive areas on palate on patient with systemic lupus erythematosis.

Fig 2-23 Rash in patient with discoid lupus erythematosis.

is important to realise that these autoantibodies are only associated with and not the cause of the condition. It is possible to have the clinical syndrome without detecting the expected antibody. Similarly it is possible to have the autoantibodies and not develop the disease.

Organ-Specific Autoimmune Diseases

A variety of other immunological conditions have oral features. Some commonly encountered are autoimmune thyroid disease, pernicious anaemia and Addison's disease:

- *Autoimmune thyroid disease* can produce both hyperthyroidism and hypothyroidism. Both are associated with few direct oral changes, but the psychological effects can be associated with occasional presentation of oral dysaesthesia or facial pain.
- *Pernicious anaemia* can result in vitamin B_{12} deficiency and, as a consequence, may produce oral symptoms such as recurrent aphthous ulceration and mucosal discomfort.
- *Addison's disease*, resulting from the autoimmune destruction of the adrenal gland, results in inadequate production of cortisol and aldosterone. Consequently, as a result of raised adrenocorticotrophic hormone (ACTH) levels, it is associated with oral mucosal pigmentation.
- *Myasthenia gravis* produces weakness of the facial muscles, characteristically worse as the day progresses.

Vasculitic-Induced Oral Disease

Vasculitis is inflammation in the walls of blood vessels, usually initiated by

Table 2-6 **Autoantibodies in systemic autoimmune conditions**

Antibody Class	Autoantibody	Main associated clinical presentations (prevalence)	Specificity for condition
Rheumatoid factor	RF	Rheumatoid arthritis (70%) and many other autoimmune diseases	low
Anti DNA antibodies	ds-DNA ss-DNA	SLE (70%) Many autoimmune diseases	high none
Extractable nuclear antigens	Sm Ro	SLE (5-50% by race) SLE (40%) Sjögren's (80%)	high low high
	La	SLE (15%) Sjögren's (50%)	low high
	Jo-1	Polymyositis (30%)	high
	Centromere	Systemic sclerosis (30%)	moderate
	Topoisomerase 1(SCL-70)	Systemic sclerosis (30%)	high
Anti phospholipid antibodies	Cardiolipin or beta2-glycoprotein	Antiphospholipid antibody syndrome/SLE (30%)	high
Anti-neutrophil cytoplasmic antibodies	pANCA/MPO	Churg-Strauss syndrome Microscopic polyangitis	moderate
	cANCA/PR3	Wegener's granulomatosis	very high

immune complex deposition from the circulation. This can lead to swelling of the vessel walls, narrowing of the lumen and eventual occlusion of the vessels with consequent infarction of the tissue supplied by that vessel.

Cranial arteritis (often referred to as 'temporal arteritis') is inflammation of the medium-sized arteries in the external carotid distribution, and consequently the effects can be widespread. Patients experience pain in the maxilla, temporal region and behind the eye. Patients may also present with 'jaw claudication' where chewing induces discomfort in the masticatory muscles due to the restricted blood flow delivering inadequate oxygen to the active muscle tissue. Many patients have tenderness to palpation over the temporal arteries, which may be enlarged, tortuous and pulsatile. A biopsy of the artery has been a definitive diagnostic tool, but as only sections of the artery are involved in the inflammatory process (skip lesions) finding normal arterial tissue does not exclude the condition. Significant rises in the plasma viscosity (PV) or erythrocyte sedimentation rate (ESR) are non-specific test findings, but in association with the clinical symptoms are usually enough evidence to start treatment. If cranial arteritis is suspected it is very important to start the patient on corticosteroid therapy quickly. This is because arterial occlusion in the external carotid branches can lead to sudden-onset and irreversible blindness due to involvement of the central retinal artery. Patients should be referred to a specialist in vascular medicine for long-term care.

Polyarteritis nodosa has an association with hepatitis B infection, although it can also arise as a drug reaction. Arterial aneurysms are seen on angiography early in the condition but eventually vessel occlusion and tissue infarction follow. The timing of effects on the oral tissues varies but the presentation is one of painful and extensive necrotic oral ulceration that is slow to heal. The multisystem effects can be more important, with neurological, renal and cardiac problems complicating patient management in dentistry.

Wegener's granulomatosis (Fig 2-24) is one of a number of conditions that are grouped together into midline granuloma syndrome. In this condition a destructive granulomatous process gradually spreads through the midface with often lethal systemic involvement. Wegener's particularly involves the respiratory tract with granulomatous change and vasculitis. In the mouth it classically produces strawberry-like swollen gingival or palatal tissue. Often this is an early feature of the disease and may allow referral for specialist care before the condition has become too advanced. When suspected, detection of the antibodies c-ANCA and PR3 in the blood can be useful confirmation but, as with all autoantibodies, they are not present in every case. Treatment is with corticosteroids and cytotoxic drugs, such as cyclophosphamide, which slow the progress of the condition.

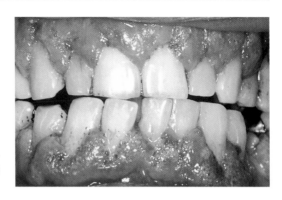

Fig 2-24 'Strawberry' gingivitis as a result of Wegner's granulomatosis.

Kawasaki disease is also known as mucocutaneous lymph node syndrome (MCLS) and usually presents in children with desquamation of the lips fingers and toes. Intraoral findings include mucosal erythema, labial oedema and a 'strawberry' tongue. Cervical lymphadenopathy is common. These features are self-limiting, but there is often involvement of the coronary arteries, where vessel-wall inflammation can lead to aneurysms, infarction and death. Patients suspected of having this condition should be immediately referred to a paediatric cardiologist. Those who have a history of Kawasaki's disease may have residual cardiac damage, and antibiotic prophylaxis may be appropriate for invasive dental procedures.

Summary

- Connective-tissue diseases or their treatments commonly have effects on the mouth and oral tissues.
- Vasculitic disorders are uncommon in the mouth but important to recognize.
- Cranial arteritis is a cause of headache or facial pain.

Further Reading

Allergy
Wray D, Rees SR, Gibson J, Forsyth A. The role of allergy in oral mucosal disease. QJM 2000;93:8,507-511.

Axell T. Hypersensitivity of the oral mucosa: clinics and pathology. Acta Odontol Scand 2001;59:5,315-319.

Lichen planus

Epstein JB, Wan LS, Gorsky M, Zhang L. Oral lichen planus: progress in understanding its malignant potential and the implications for clinical management. Oral Surg Oral Med Oral Pathol Oral Radiol Endod 2003;96:1,32-37.

Carrozzo M, Gandolfo S. Oral diseases possibly associated with hepatitis C virus. Crit Rev Oral Biol Med 2003;14:2,115-127.

Recurrent oral ulceration

Scully C, Gorsky M, Lozada-Nur F. The diagnosis and management of recurrent aphthous stomatitis: a consensus approach. J Am Dent Assoc 2003;134:2,200-207.

Calabrese L, Fleischer AB. Thalidomide: current and potential clinical applications. Am J Med. 2000;108:6,487-495.

Vesiculobullous disease

Challacombe SJ, Setterfield J, Shirlaw P et al. Immunodiagnosis of pemphigus and mucous membrane pemphigoid. Acta Odontol Scand 2001;59:4,226-234.

Systemic autoimmune disease

Johnsson R, Moen K, Vestrheim D, Szodoray P. Current issues in Sjogren's syndrome. Oral Dis 2002;8:3,130-140.

De Rossi SS, Glick M. Lupus erythematosus: considerations for dentistry. J Am Dent Assoc 1998;129:3,330-339.

Chapter 3

Lumps and Bumps

Aim

The aim of this chapter is to describe those oral or perioral lesions that present as a lump or swelling.

Outcome

After reading this chapter you should have an understanding of the various oral and perioral lumps and swellings, their diagnosis and management.

Vascular Anomalies (Figs 3-1 to 3-6)

Haemangioma

Haemangiomas are generally regarded as hamartomatous and as such are developmental in origin. A number do appear however to arise later in life and may represent benign neoplasms. The lesions are generally red or bluish/purple in colour and of soft consistency. They tend to be either flat or raised but typically blanch on pressure. Clinically they are divided, depending on vessel type, into either capillary haemangiomas (port wine stain) or cavernous haemangiomas, although it is not unusual to have combinations of both. In addition to involving the soft tissues they may extend into underlying bone or salivary glands. It is not unusual for the appearance

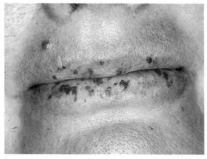

Fig 3-1 Hereditary haemorrhagic telangiectasia affecting the lips.

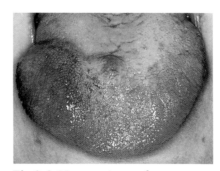

Fig 3-2 Haemangioma of tongue.

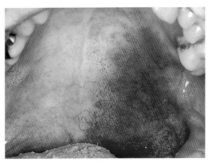

Fig 3-3 Capillary haemangioma affecting the palate.

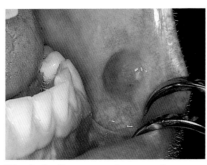

Fig 3-4 Cavernous haemangioma on the buccal mucosa.

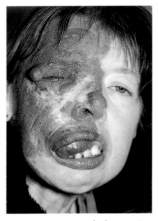

Fig 3-5 Trigemino-encephalo-angiomatosis (Sturge-Weber syndrome).

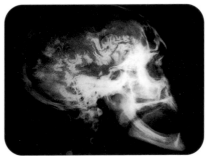

Fig 3-6 Lateral skull radiograph of patient with Sturge-Weber syndrome demonstrating calcification of the leptomeninges.

on the surface to be related to a much deeper underlying vascular anomaly, which makes surgical removal difficult. Generally these lesions are of cosmetic significance only. Treatment, if required, usually involves cryotherapy or laser ablation, but in some more extensive lesions a feeder vessel can be blocked using an intravascular procedure, which may diminish the size of the anomaly.

Sturge -Weber Syndrome (Trigemino-Encephaloangiomatosis)

This congenital disorder comprises a combination of haemangiomatous lesions affecting the face and also the ipsilateral leptomeninges. Apart from the facial disfigurement these patients frequently suffer from epilepsy. The abnormal cerebral vessels may become calcified and, as a consequence, visible radiographically.

Hereditary Haemorrhagic Telangiectasia
This disorder is transmitted as an autosomal dominant and comprises multiple small collections of dilated capillaries (telangiectases), which are found predominantly on the face, lips, mouth, nasal tissues and intestinal mucosa. Recurrent nosebleeds are common and there is also a risk of gastrointestinal haemorrhage. As a consequence patients may become iron-deficient. Treatment is usually symptomatic, with either laser or cryotherapy ablation of problematic telangiectasias.

Varicosities
Varicose veins are commonly seen on the ventrolateral sides of the tongue and occasionally the lower lip, particularly in the elderly. These are of no particular significance, although those on the lower lip may give rise to cosmetic concern and can be treated locally with cryotherapy.

Malignant Vascular Swellings
These are rare anomalies and can occur on the oral mucosa, such as Kaposi's sarcoma in patients with HIV infection.

Lymphangioma
These lesions are not dissimilar to haemangiomas, except they consist of lymph vessels. As a consequence the swellings are usually not discoloured or have a slightly translucent appearance. Most are present at birth and require no specific treatment. A variant is the cystic hygroma, which is a lymphangiomatous malformation that affects the head and more frequently the neck, producing a visible mass, noticeable either at birth or shortly after. This may require surgical removal.

Connective Tissue Hyperplasias (Figs 3-7 to 3-10)
This group of disorders are a result of a localised excess production of fibrous tissue. They can be either developmental or, more commonly, acquired. The acquired variants most frequently present as lobulated swellings to which the term polyp or occasionally granuloma is applied. A variety of terms describing such polyps is used depending on their site, such as fibrous epulis* on the gingiva or fibroepithelial polyp on other sites of the oral mucosa. Those lesions

*(* epulis is a generic term used for a 'lump' on the gingiva)*

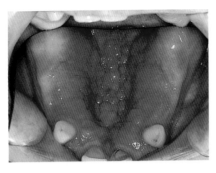

Fig 3-7 Papillary hyperplasia of the palate associated with a mild denture stomatitis.

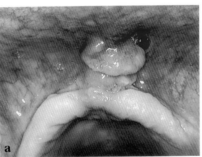
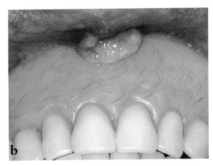

Fig 3-8 (a) Denture related irritation hyperplasia; (b) denture in place.

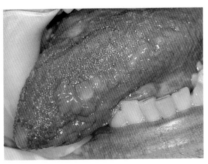
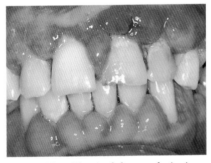

Fig 3-9 Multiple small fibroepithelial polyps on the tongue. This appearance can be associated with Cowden's syndrome. A rare, inherited, disorder associated with malignant disease, particularly carcinomas of breast, thyroid and colon.

Fig 3-10 Gingival hyperplasia in a patient taking nifedipine.

associated with the peripherary of an ill-fitting denture are termed denture irritation hyperplasias, whereas multiple fibrous nodules not infrequently seen under the fitting surface of a denture, often in association with denture stomatitis, are termed papillary hyperplasia of the palate. All these lesions represent a reaction to local irritation. Generally, once the irritation is removed there will be some regression, although they rarely completely resolve.

Treatment, if required, involves removing the irritation, where possible, and surgical excision.

Pyogenic granuloma (Fig 3-11)

This reddish-coloured lesion comprises of a 'lump' of granulation tissue, often with an ulcerated surface covered by a yellowish fibrinous exudate, and

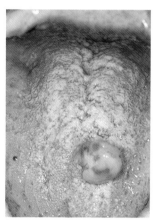

Fig 3-11 Pyogenic granuloma of tongue – note the vascular appearance of this ulcerated lesion covered by a fibrinous exudate.

can occur anywhere on the oral mucosa or skin, usually following trauma. Those occurring on the gingiva are usually termed a vascular epulis, although the aetiology is probably identical to those presenting at other sites. Their relatively sudden appearance and often dramatic rate of growth means that they may need to be differentiated from a neoplasm, and treatment is generally surgical excision. It is essential to remove any underlying irritation for those occurring on the gingiva, such as overhanging restorations, foreign bodies or calculus to prevent recurrence.

Pregnancy Epulis

This lesion is identical to a vascular epulis (pyogenic granuloma), except it occurs during pregnancy, most frequently towards the end of the first trimester. After pregnancy it may regress spontaneously or decrease in size. As a consequence surgical intervention can be left until after the birth of the child unless the lesion becomes bothersome, although oral hygiene measures to remove local irritation should be instituted.

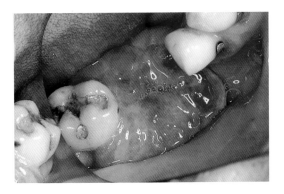

Fig 3-12 Peripheral giant cell granuloma on the lower alveolar ridge. Such a lesion may mimic an oral carcinoma, and a similar appearance may be seen with a central giant cell granuloma and in hyperparathyroidism.

Peripheral Giant Cell Granuloma (Giant Cell Epulis) (Fig 3-12)

This relatively uncommon gingival swelling usually develops from the premolar region forwards and presents as a purplish/brown lesion. Growth is often rapid and may be mistaken for a malignancy. Treatment is surgical excision, and the characteristic histology will determine the diagnosis. This appearance can also occur as a result of a lesion more central in the bone erupting out onto the gingiva. This is the central giant cell granuloma, which requires surgical curettage. These conditions need to be differentiated from a similar presentation that can arise as a feature of hyperparathyroidism. As a consequence the histopathological diagnosis of giant cell granuloma usually requires further investigation including:

- radiographs – to identify a more central lesion
- serum calcium - elevated in hyperparathyroidism
- serum parathyroid hormone (PTH) levels.

Hyperparathyroidism

Hyperparathyroidism can produce an intra-oral lesion known as a brown tumour. It presents orally as described above for giant cell granuloma. It can either arise through a parathyroid adenoma (primary) or as a result of a reactive change secondary to chronic renal damage (renal osteodystrophy). Management of this condition should tackle the underlying cause.

Chronic Hyperplastic Gingivitis

Fibrous enlargement of the gingiva can arise as a result of a florid reaction to plaque-induced gingivitis. It is more commonly seen in adolescents and those with a tendency to mouth-breathing. It usually responds to local oral hygiene measures.

A similar appearance can occur as a developmental anomaly, hereditary gingival fibromatosis. This is often transmitted through an autosomal dominant gene, although sporadic cases are not unknown. Management involves meticulous oral hygiene but also some repeated removal of the excess gingival tissue.

Enlarged fibrous tuberosities are probably a variant of hereditary gingival fibromatosis. Management depends on any associated problems, including difficulty with maintaining an acceptable level of oral hygiene or the fitting of a prosthesis, when the excess tissue may need to be reduced.

Drug-Induced Gingival Hyperplasia
This condition presents with bulbous fibrous gingival hyperplasia and represents an exaggerated response to plaque in patients taking phenytoin, ciclosporin A, nifedipine or occasionally other calcium channel-blocking drugs. Management involves either changing the medication or, more importantly, maintaining scrupulous oral hygiene, which may prevent its development. In some instances surgical reduction of the excess gingival tissue may be required.

Benign Mucosal Neoplasia
Benign neoplasms can arise from any of the tissues comprising the oral mucosa.

Squamous Cell Papilloma (Fig 3-13)
This slow-growing lesion resembles a small cauliflower with frond-like processes and can arise at any site on the oral epithelium. Its colour can vary from normal mucosa through to white, depending on the degree of associated keratinisation. In many instances these lesions are of viral aetiology associated with the human papilloma virus. Treatment consists of surgical excision.

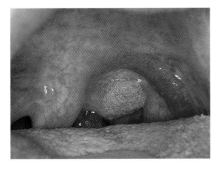

Fig 3-13 Squamous cell papilloma in the oropharynx. Such "cauliflower" lesions may be pink or white depending on the degree of associated keratinisation.

43

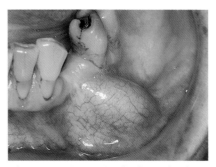

Fig 3-14 Lipoma in the buccal sulcus. Note the slightly yellowish tinge to this lesion, which, although asymptomatic, may be easily mistaken for a dental abscess.

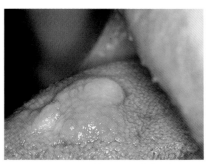

Fig 3-15 Neurofibroma of the dorsum of tongue in patient with neurofibromatosis.

Lipoma (Fig 3-14)

These usually present as slow-growing, soft, occasionally lobulated swellings, which may have a slight yellowish appearance. They are relatively common subcutaneous tumours but can also occur in the oral tissues. Those arising in the buccal sulci may be mistaken for abscesses. Treatment is usually surgical excision.

Neurofibroma (Fig 3-15)

Neurofibroma may present as a solitary nodule, similar to a fibroepithelial polyp, and as a consequence is usually differentiated by histology. Neurofibromatosis (von Recklinghausen's disease) is a developmental disorder of multiple neurofibromas affecting the skin as well as the oral tissues and is associated with patchy light-brown melanotic pigmentation (café-au-lait spots). In many instances this condition is hereditary. Malignant transformation in the neurofibromas can occur in 5-15% of cases, and as a consequence the condition requires monitoring.

Multiple Endocrine Neoplasia Syndrome (MEN)

Multiple neuromas on the oral mucosa are an important feature of MEN-type IIB. This inherited syndrome is associated with Marfanoid features and medullary carcinoma of the thyroid, which may develop in adolescence. Phaeochromocytoma, which is a tumour of the adrenal glands, also occurs. The presence of the oral mucosal neuromas may precede the development of endocrine neoplasia, and as a consequence its early detection is essential and relevant endocrine monitoring undertaken.

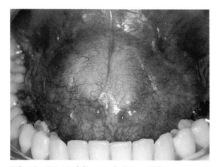

Fig 3-16 Sublingual dermaid cyst.

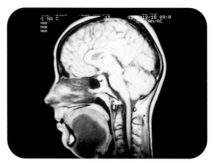

Fig 3-17 The full extent of this lesion as demonstrated on sagittal MR scan (T1weighted).

Miscellaneous Oral Soft-Tissue Swellings

Foliate Papillitis

Foliate papillae are often associated with lingual tonsillar tissue and are typically found on the posterior lateral margins of the tongue. Swelling of this tissue can arise as a result of trauma from teeth or dentures or as a reactive (inflammatory) hyperplasia of the lymphoid tissue. The swelling and appearance at this site of the tongue can give cause for concern and consequently it may be surgically removed. Removal of any underlying cause may also produce resolution.

Sublingual Dermoid (Epidermoid) Cysts

These are uncommon causes of swelling in the midline floor of mouth/sublingual area and are of developmental origin. Their presence may go unrecognised for a considerable time and can result in a fairly prominent swelling expanding into the submental/submandibular region. The condition needs to be differentiated from a plunging ranula, and treatment involves surgical removal (Figs 3-16 and 3-17).

Bone Anomalies

There are a large number of conditions that affect bone, but only those that are likely to be referred for an oral medicine opinion will be considered here.

Exostosis and Tori

An exostosis is a term used to describe a bony outgrowth that may have either

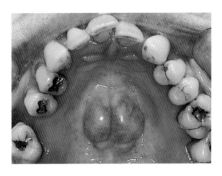

Fig 3-18 Torus palatinus.

a developmental or reactive origin. It is usually of no clinical significance and treatment is rarely indicated.

Tori

Tori are exostoses that occur at characteristic sites. In the palate (torus palatinus) they are midline and can either be solitary or multiple (Fig 3-18). In the mandible (torus mandibularis) these are on the lingual surface adjacent to the premolar teeth, where they present as either a solitary or multiple dome-shaped swellings (Fig 3-19). The exact aetiology of this condition is unknown, although it does occur at the sites of maximal functional stress for these bones and may represent a reactive response to this.

In most cases no specific treatment is required, although patients frequently become concerned as to the nature of tori, as attention is usually drawn to them following trauma to the overlying mucosa. They can be removed surgically if they interfere with denture construction or stability.

Osteoma

An osteoma is a benign neoplasm of bone that usually occurs as a solitary, slow-growing nodule. Treatment, if required, consists of surgical removal. Multiple osteomas of the jaws may occur as a component of Gardner's syndrome, which is a hereditary disorder associated with polyposis coli. The significance of this condition is the pre-malignant potential of the polyps, which will require careful monitoring. This syndrome may be also associated with multiple fibrous skin nodules and sebaceous cysts.

Osteosarcoma

Osteosarcoma is a primary malignant neoplasm of bone, which fortunately is rare in the jaws. The presentation is frequently of a fairly rapidly enlarg-

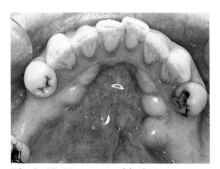

Fig 3-19 Torus mandibularis.

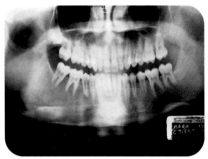

Fig 3-20 Diffuse, expansile lesion with classic ground glass appearance in patient with fibrous dysplasia affecting right mandible.

ing swelling that may be accompanied by pain, loss of sensation and loosening of the overlying teeth. The radiographic appearance is somewhat variable but classically includes a sunray pattern of bone deposition. However, definitive diagnosis is histological and the management of the primary condition is surgical removal.

Osteosarcoma can develop in association with Paget's disease of the bone (see below) or following radiotherapy to the area.

Fibro-Osseous Lesions of the Jaws

There are a number of conditions that can be either developmental or benign neoplasms involving the fibro-osseous components of bone. Most are relatively rare and unlikely to present to a dental clinic.

Cherubism

Cherubism is a rare autosomal dominant inherited dysplasia of bone presenting in early childhood as symmetrical, painless swellings of the jaws, giving a characteristic 'cherubic' appearance that subsides during adolescence.

Fibrous Dysplasia (Fig 3-20)

This condition can affect either one bone (monostotic) or several bones (polyostotic) and presents most frequently during adolescence as a slow-growing expansion of the affected bone, the growth of which ceases during early adulthood.

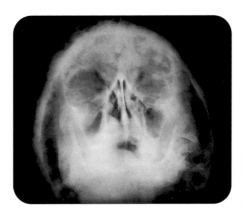

Fig 3-21 Paget's disease of bone. Skull radiograph demonstrates cotton wool appearance and loss of normal architecture of affected bone.

A variation of polyostotic fibrous dysplasia is Albright syndrome, in which the bone lesions are associated with melanotic pigmented patches of the skin (café-au-lait spots), precocious puberty in females and occasionally other endocrine abnormalities.

Diagnosis

The above conditions are usually diagnosed by a combination of clinical, characteristic radiological and histological appearances and serum chemistry. The latter may reveal an elevation of alkaline phosphatase during an active phase of the lesion but will otherwise be within normal limits.

Treatment

In most cases these conditions require no specific treatment as further development stops once growth ceases and certainly treatment should be deferred until then. At that time surgical correction of any deformity can be undertaken.

Paget's Disease of Bone

This relatively common condition predominantly affects people over 40 with an incidence of approximately 3%. It is particularly common among those of Anglo-Saxon origin. The condition is of unknown aetiology, although a 'slow virus', possibly a paramyxovirus, has been suggested.

The commonest sites affected are the femur, pelvis, tibia, skull and spine, although any bone can be involved. Most cases are asymptomatic but features include:
• pain in the affected bone or joints

- deformity, with bowing of the leg bones and flattening of the skull ('Tam O'Shanter hat' appearance)
- complications due to nerve compression such as deafness
- fracture through abnormal bone with associated poor healing
- development of osteosarcoma (rare).

Paget's disease is essentially a disorder of bone remodelling with uncontrolled bone turnover that results radiographically in loss of the normal bony architecture and a cotton wool appearance (Fig 3-21).

Diagnosis

This condition is often a chance discovery on clinical or radiographic examination. However, the finding of increased serum alkaline phosphatase with normal serum calcium and phosphate reflecting increased bone turnover is a typical biochemical feature. Histology is often not required but would reveal a characteristic pattern of erratic bone resorption and desposition.

Treatment

In a number of cases Paget's disease does not require treatment, although the increased bone turnover can be controlled using calcitonin or diphosphonates. It is of note that difficulty may be encountered with dental extractions due to the presence of associated hypercementosis of the roots.

Conclusions

- Lumps, bumps and swellings of the oral and perioral tissues are common.
- Most of this group of lesions are benign.
- Many of these lesions are clinically similar and need to be differentiated histologically.
- Occasionally some of these lesions are an oral manifestation of a more general problem and further investigation is required.

Further Reading

Soames JV, Southam JC. Oral Pathology 4th ed. Oxford: Oxford University Press, 2005.

Chapter 4
Infections of the Oral Mucosa

Aim

This chapter reviews the common oral mucosal and facial infections.

Outcome

After reading this chapter you should be familiar with the presenting features, investigations and management strategy for commonly encountered oro-facial infections.

Introduction

Infections of the oral mucosa are fall into three broad categories.
• bacterial
• viral
• fungal.

Some take short-term advantage of a compromised immune system and others become chronic problems. When presented with an infection in clinical practice, in addition to consideration of the infecting organism, it is important that the circumstances of the infection are taken into account. This allows local, systemic or environmental factors to be identified and managed. A principle of managing infections is that treatment should follow identification of the active organism and its sensitivity to antimicrobial therapy. Close liaison with the microbiologist will ensure that appropriate samples are taken and properly transported to the laboratory. Antimicrobial therapy is not required for every patient. In many cases attention to local factors, such as the removal of an abscessed tooth, is all that is needed.

Bacterial Infections

Bacterial infections of the face and oral mucosa usually present as acute problems. They often represent local alterations in the host-bacterial balance, changing a commensal into a pathogen. Bacterial conditions seen include:
• acute ulcerative gingivitis (Fig 4-1)

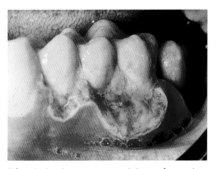

Fig 4-1 Acute necrotising ulcerative gingivitis (ANUG). The presentation of this condition warrants further investigation for possible underlying immunosuppression.

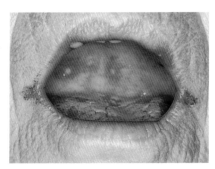

Fig 4-2 Aphthous type ulceration affecting the palate and tongue, with in addition bilateral angular cheilitis in a patient with vitamin B_{12} deficiency.

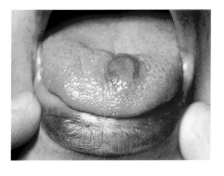

Fig 4-3 Primary syphilitic chancre on the dorsum of the tongue.

- facial abscess
- staphylococcal and streptococcal infections
  - bacterial mucositis
  - angular cheilitis (Fig 4-2)
  - impetigo
  - erysipelas
- syphilis (Fig 4-3)
- tuberculosis.

Acute Ulcerative Gingivitis

Acute ulcerative gingivitis is a necrotising condition of the marginal gingival tissues, seen mostly in smokers during the winter months. It is usually localised to the anterior gingivae and, as well as being painful, it also gives the patient a very unpleasant characteristic odour. In the immunocompromised the lesions may be found in any part of the dental arch and be much more extensive. In extreme cases they extend to include bone as well as soft-tissue necrosis. The cause is an anaerobic fuso-spirocheatal complex that is sensitive to metronidazole (200mg three times daily for seven days). Oral hygiene measures and topical use of chlorhexidine are often all that are required in the less severe cases in an immunocompetent host.

Facial Abscess

Facial abscesses are most commonly of dental origin and present with a swelling over the body or angle of the mandible or the infra-orbital region in patients who typically have dental neglect. If untreated, the infection will discharge onto the facial skin, producing an unsightly appearance and a persisting facial scar. The pattern of the discharge from a dental abscess to the skin or the mouth will depend on the position of the tooth roots relative to muscle insertions. Gravity then works to make most swellings from the upper teeth appear over the lower face and from the lower teeth either at the border of the mandible or the sublingual or submental area of the anterior neck. These are mixed infections of anaerobes and aerobes and require removal of the cause (extraction or pulpectomy) and, following culture and sensitivity assessment of a drained pus sample, a course of antibiotics may be provided to augment surgical management. Antibiotic therapy is not an alternative but is a supportive therapy. On rare occasions culture will suggest actinomycosis. Actinomyces species are common commensals in the mouth, but a true infection is uncommon.

Streptococcal and Staphylococcal Infections
Mucositis

Staphylococci are occasionally implicated in mucosal infection, particularly in the palate beneath dentures. The erythematous change is not clinically distinguishable from that produced by a chronic candidal infection and reinforces the need for microbiological investigation as part of the process used to reduce denture-induced stomatitis. Denture and oral hygiene measures are usually all that are required to settle the problem, which is mostly asymptomatic. Systemic antibiotics are rarely used.

Angular Cheilitis

This is a multifactorial problem. Systemic factors, such as iron deficiency or diabetes mellitus, act with local factors, such as a reduction in the facial vertical height due to a worn prosthesis, to allow staphylococci and candidal organisms to become established and pathogenic at the corners of the mouth. Management should address all issues, including correction of systemic factors, facial height and appliance hygiene. Often no more is required, but

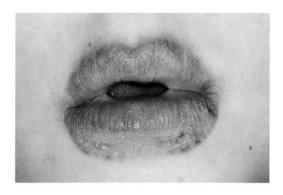

Fig 4-4 Lick eczema. Note how the area of inflammation extends as far as the tongue can reach. Occasionally this condition can become secondarily infected with *Staphylococcous aureus* to produce golden-coloured crusting.

when the problem persists the use of an agent with both antifungal and antibacterial actions, such as miconazole, is preferred. Where the skin inflammation has been long-standing, the use of miconazole with hydrocortisone cream allows the skin architecture to return to normal by eliminating persisting inflammation. Abnormal skin is rapidly recolonised by the pathogens, and the angular cheilitis returns quickly.

Perioral Skin Infections (Fig 4-4)
Perioral skin infections are common in children and people who are immunocompromised. Impetigo is caused by *Staphylococcus aureus*, beta haemolytic streptococci or both. The staphylococci tend to produce thin-walled blisters, whereas a more crusting form tends to be associated with streptococci. Multiple lesions may present around the face but each area of impetigo remains discrete. It can spread rapidly to other individuals in close contact with the patient. Often the appearance can suggest recurrent herpes simplex to those unfamiliar with impetigo, and it is entirely possible that the skin breach initiated by herpes simplex may allow the entry of the impetigo organisms in some cases. Although a rare complication, an acute glomerulonephiritis may follow, in common with other streptococcal infections. Erysipelas is streptococcal in origin and the organism usually gains entry through an existing skin breach. It presents as a spreading erythematous facial infection with a well-defined advancing edge. The patient is usually systemically unwell and responds rapidly to penicillin treatment.

Syphilis
Although in decline for many years, syphilis and its oral manifestations are again becoming more common. The infecting organism is *Tremonema pallidum*, and there are oral features in all three stages. These are:

- the primary chancre
- 'snail-track' ulcers of the secondary stage
- the gumma or leukoplakia of the tertiary stage.

Few practitioners have seen this condition nowadays, which makes diagnosis difficult. A high degree of suspicion and good laboratory collaboration is essential.

Tuberculosis

As with syphilis, the incidence of tuberculosis is on the rise, particularly in the immunosuppressed and immigrant populations. The common causative organism is *Mycobacterium tuberculosis*. In the immunocompromised host atypical mycobacteria may be responsible for infections, and it has been suggested that *Mycobacterium paratuberculosis* may be involved in Crohn's disease and orofacial granulomatosis. In patients with active tuberculosis oral involvement is rare, but the organisms can produce enlarged cervical lymph nodes, an oropharyngeal abscess or a chronic ulcer on the tongue. Biopsy of a suspected lesion is essential to confirm the diagnosis, finding the tubercle bacilli in a chronic granulomatous reaction. Identification of a patient with tuberculosis requires notification to the public health services to identify, trace and screen any contacts of the patient and thus limit spread of the disease.

Viral Infections (Figs 4-5 to 4-8)

In the orofacial region, viral infections, particularly with the herpes group of viruses, are very frequent. The clinical problems encountered are given in Table 4-1.

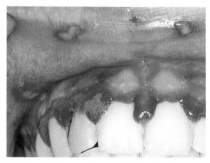

Fig 4-5 Primary herpetic gingival stomatitis.

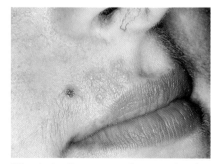

Fig 4-6 Recurrent herpes simplex lesion of the upper lip (cold sore). In this instance the lesion is at a relatively early vesicular phase.

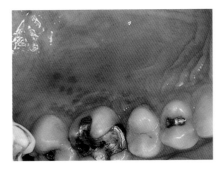

Fig 4-7 Recurrent herpes simplex infection of the palate.

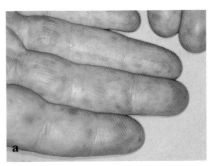

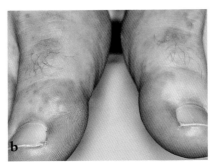

Fig 4-8 Vesicular lesions of the fingers (a) and toes (b) in a patient with hand, foot and mouth disease.

Table 4-1 **Herpes viruses in orofacial disease**

- Herpes viruses
  - HHV1 & 2   *Acute gingivostomatitis, herpes labialis*
  - HHV3   *Chickenpox, shingles (zoster)*
  - HHV4   *Glandular fever*
  - HHV5   *Cytomegalovirus ulceration/retinitis (immunocompromised)*

- Coxsackie viruses   *Hand, foot and mouth disease, herpangina*
- Paramyxoviruses   *Mumps*
- HIV   *Oral effects of immunsuppression*
- Human papilloma virus   *Viral papilloma, oral cancer*

Herpes Group Viruses

At present eight human herpes viruses (HHV) are described. However, herpes viruses 6, 7 and 8 do not seem to directly cause any oral infections. HHV 8 is, however, found in Kaposi's sarcoma, but its exact role in this condition is unclear. HHV 6 is associated with a maculopapular rash termed Exanthem subitum in infants. HHV 1-5 all produce limited diseases in healthy adults, both as primary infections and, in some, reactivations. In the very young, elderly and immunocompromised, however, life-threatening disseminated infections can result. Evidence of infection in these groups requires prompt systemic treatment. It is important to remember that in immunocompromised hosts these viral conditions often present in atypical ways. A high degree of suspicion is usually required to make the clinical diagnosis.

HHV 1 and 2 – Herpes Simplex 1 and 2

These viruses are the classical 'herpes' viruses, producing acute herpetic gingivostomatitis and recurrent herpes simplex ('cold sores'). As with all of the herpes group, the virus can be acquired without the typical primary seroconversion illness. This is particularly the case in younger children. In all patients with acute gingivostomatitis there is systemic malaise, fever and cervical lymphadenopathy together with widespread oral ulceration, affecting attached and reflected mucosa, and lip-crusting. It is important that the patient's fluid intake is maintained during this acute phase. In most children the condition will resolve in seven to 10 days, and by the time of presentation there is little benefit in systemic antiviral therapy except in the immunocompromised. Adults, however, can have a significant illness. This can extend to some weeks, and early antiviral therapy such as famciclovir 750mg daily for seven days is appropriate. On rare occasions the virus will disseminate and a herpes simplex encephalopathy with residual neurological deficit may result.

About one-third of patients with serological exposure to herpes simplex virus will experience periodic reactivation. Recurrent herpes simplex lesions can affect any part of the trigeminal distribution, but common sites are the skin around the mouth and nose and the palatal mucosa. Most often there is a trigger for the reactivation of the viral symptoms. This varies from person to person, but can be a concomitant systemic illness, sunlight, menstruation and stressful life events. The herpetic lesions are intraepithelial vesicles that quickly rupture and crust, often lasting about 10 days from onset to resolution. It remains unclear whether there is a role for topical antiviral medication in the uncomplicated recurrent herpes simplex lesion. Some patients are troubled with almost continuous 'recurrent' herpetic lesions, however, and for them 200mg twice-daily prophylaxis with aciclovir can be very useful. Similarly, some patients get very extensive facial lesions with recurrent HSV and these, although intermittent, can be very disabling. Again systemic aciclovir (200mg five times daily for seven days) is appropriate at the onset of symptoms in these patients.

HHV 3 – Varicella Zoster

This virus is responsible for 'chickenpox' during the seroconversion illness and zoster on reactivation. Chickenpox causes fever and malaise together with a vesicular rash from which the vesicles dry and crust. They are intensely itchy. The virus is spread by direct contact with the vesicles from an infected individual. Intraoral ulceration is seen in some individuals but it is much less marked and severe that that seen in HHV1 and 2. Most patients recover from the initial illness without incident.

Recurrent varicella zoster is termed shingles. As with herpes simplex this reactivation usually affects only one dermatome, but any part of the body, face trunk or limbs can be involved. Unlike herpes simplex, however, it is associated with significant neuropathic nerve damage, and persisting pain during and after the reactivation (post-herpetic neuralgia) is common. Zoster is best treated with a systemic antiviral such as famciclovir. If pain persists after the reactivation has cleared then standard measures for treating neuropathic pain, such as tricyclic drugs, can be used to good effect.

HHV 4 – Epstein-Barr Virus

This virus is responsible for glandular fever as its seroconversion illness. No recurrent problems have been identified. HHV 4 has been found, however, in the epithelial cells in oral hairy leukoplakia and it seems to have a predilection for salivary tissue. Burkitt's lymphoma and nasopharyngeal carcinoma are known to be associated with this virus in some ethnic groups. There is increasing evidence that HHV 4 is linked to the development of lymphomas, particularly in the immunocompromised patient.

Glandular fever presents in older children with fever, general malaise and cervical lymphadenopathy. Intraoral ulceration and rash on the palate are found in differing degrees from individual to individual. No antiviral drug is currently very effective in the management of this virus. Thus glandular fever is managed with supportive care, with the patient maintaing a good fluid intake and using appropriate antipyretic analgesics.

HHV 5 - Cytomegalovirus

This virus is found on serological testing in about 50% of adults. However, in the healthy adult there is neither a recognised seroconversion illness nor a recurring problem. In the immunocompromised person this virus can be lethal with disseminated infection, retinal infection with consequent blindness and superficial erosions or herpetic type ulceration in the mouth. In these patients systemic treatment with ganciclovir or foscarnet remains the most helpful therapy, but this is not always successful.

Coxsackie Viruses

Coxsackie A virus subtypes are associated with herpangina (A2,4,5,6,8) and hand, foot and mouth disease (A16) in humans. Herpangina is predominantly seen in children and produces multiple small ulcers at the back of the mouth, tonsil, uvula and pharyngeal region. These settle in a few days, and no specific treatment is required. Hand, foot and mouth disease is a highly contagious condition producing oral ulceration together with vesicles and ulcers on the palms of the hands and soles of the feet. It causes a variable degree of systemic upset and settles within two weeks in most cases. No antiviral drugs in common use have any role in coxsackie virus treatment.

Paramyxoviruses

Mumps virus belongs to the paramyxovirus group and prior to use of the MMR vaccine was a common infection in children (see Chapter 8). There is no treatment at present for paramyxovirus infections.

Human Immunodeficiency Virus (Figs 4-9 to 4-11)

Infection with HIV may be asymptomatic, but some patients experience a seroconversion illness not dissimilar to HSV1. The virus gives no direct oral lesions, but instead has many oral manifestations through the immune defi-

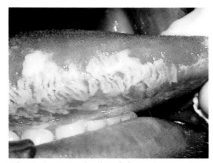

Fig 4-9 Hairy leukoplakia – in a patient with advanced human immuno-deficiency virus infection (HIV).

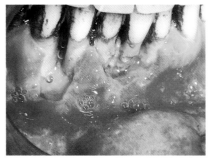

Fig 4-10 HIV-related periodontal disease. Note the relatively localised, but severe, bone loss.

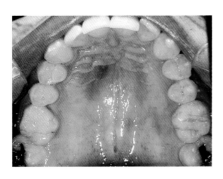

Fig 4-11 Early Kaposi's sarcoma of the hard palate in a patient with HIV.

ciency it produces. Oral manifestations associated with HIV infection include Kaposi's sarcoma, hairy leukoplakia, acute pseudomembranous oral candidiasis and lymphoma. In addition, any of the other viral conditions discussed in this chapter are likely to become significant problems, especially the herpes group viruses.

Human Papilloma Viruses (HPV)

These viruses are most associated in the orofacial region with viral papilloma formation (warts). Evidence from their role in cervical cancer as well as genital warts has led to the realisation that this virus group is likely to be involved in the development of squamous carcinomas in the mouth. Oral warts are associated with HPV subtypes 2 and 4 and focal epithelial hyperplasia with subtypes 13 and 32. Cervical cancer is associated with subtypes 16 and 18, but while the association with oral cancer remains to be determined subtypes 16, 32, 33 and 38 may be implicated.

Fungal Infections

Fungal infections in the mouth are predominantly caused by *Candida albicans* (Figs 4-12 and 4-13). In the tropics or in travellers recently returned from such areas, other fungal infections are seen, such as histoplasmosis, paracoccidioides and mucormycosis. These are systemic infections often presenting with sloughing oral ulceration and pain.

Candidal Infections

Candidal organisms involved in oral disease are predominantly *C. albicans* but others, such as *C. tropicalis*, *C. glabrata*, *C. parapsilosis* and *C. krusei*, may be causative. Oral conditions commonly associated with candida include:
- pseudomembranous candidiasis (PMC)
- chronic hyperplastic candidiasis

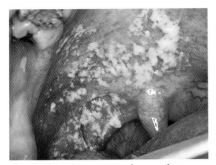

Fig 4-12 Acute pseudomembranous candidiasis affecting the soft palate and oropharynx. This presentation is not uncommon in patients using steroid-based inhalers and failing to rinse the mouth afterwards.

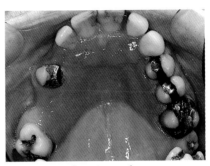

Fig 4-13 Chronic erythematous candidiasis (denture stomatitis). The area of erythema delineates the fitting surface of, in this case, an acrylic-based partial denture.

- angular cheilitis
- erythematous candidiasis.

Pseudomembranous Candidiasis

This condition is the classical candida infection 'thrush'. It is seen only when the local or systemic immune system is compromised. This may be found in poorly controlled diabetes mellitus, inhaled corticosteroid use for asthma or in HIV. Making a diagnosis of pseudomembranous candidiasis should always trigger the clinician to consider why this lesion has developed and arrange suitable investigations or therapy. At the extremes of life, however, the immune system is poorly functional and so PMC may be found without any other compromising factors. The lesions are white raised plaques that can be removed from the mucosal surface, leaving a red, inflamed surface. Typically the lesions are on the posterior palate and dorsum of the tongue. In the severely immunocompromised PMC can involve the entire mouth, pharynx and oesophagus, leading to significant dysphagia. Management should first be to correct any underlying health problem, including correct instruction in the use of steroid inhalers. Using a space device with the inhaler and rinsing the mouth after activation can significantly reduce the deposition of steroid powder on the oral and pharyngeal mucosa. Systemic antifungals such as fluconazole and itraconazole are to be preferred for treating PMC and produce significant effects within 48 hours. Prolonged use to treat recurrent PMC in HIV-positive and other systemically immunocompromised patients does lead to emergence of resistant organisms. Specialist advice should be sought when treating these patient groups.

Chronic Hyperplastic Candidiasis

This condition was previously referred to as a 'candidal leukoplakia'. The lesion is indistinguishable from many other idiopathic white lesions of the mucosa. The histological appearance indicates candidal invasion of the upper layers of the epithelium. It is unclear whether this is a cause of the lesion or an opportunistic invasion of altered mucosa, as can be seen in some patients with lichen planus. There is often a degree of dysplasia in the tissue. As in lichen planus (Chapter 2) this change seems related to the invading organisms, as treatment with systemic antifungals often reverses the histological appearance. Chronic hyperplastic candidal lesions are suspected of having a higher malignant transformation rate than normal mucosa and so should be kept under long-term review. Biopsies should be performed if any morphological changes occur. It is important to address risk factors, such as smoking and alcohol use, in patients with chronic hyperplastic candidiasis.

Angular Cheilitis

Angular cheilitis is often a mixed infective picture with candida and staphylococci. This condition is covered in the bacterial infections section above.

Erythematous Candidiasis

This is the picture most often seen beneath a denture or appliance where red mucosa is often found. It can also be triggered by prolonged broad-spectrum antibiotic use. In some patients minor forms seem to be present without obvious cause. The spectrum of erythematous candidiasis extends from small discrete red lesions on the palatal mucosa to the irritated and inflamed picture covering the entire denture-bearing area, commonly referred to as 'denture stomatitis'. It can also include changes elsewhere in the mouth, such as the erythematous tongue seen in patients with end-stage Sjögren's syndrome. These lesions seem to arise because of local rather than systemic factors. Treatment should be based around local oral and appliance hygiene and reducing dietary carbohydrate intake. Despite this, small areas of erythema persist in some patients. It is sensible to accept these asymptomatic areas, as they are of no clinical consequence. Topical antifungals have a very limited role to play in the management of erythematous candidiasis and are not a substitute for good hygiene practice.

Chronic Mucocutaneous Candidiasis

This condition reflects a variety of systemic problems that result in an individual's immune system failing to form an adequate immune response to candida. The clinical picture is variable, but the patient usually presents with chronic nail, skin and oral problems in differing degrees. Often there are other associated features, such as iron deficiency, haematological and endocrine abnormalities. The oral candidal lesions are difficult to manage, but in most patients they are chronic hyperplastic candidiasis and therefore asymptomatic. The malignant potential remains, however, and careful follow-up is required.

Summary

- Infections suggest a breakdown in the host/parasite balance – it is important to find out why this has occurred.
- Antimicrobial therapy is not an alternative to adequate local or systemic health measures, including surgical drainage of infection.

Further reading

General oral microbiology
Bagg, McFarlane, Poxton et al. Essentials of Microbiology for Dental Students. Oxford: Oxford University Press.

Clarkson JE, Worthington HV, Eden OB. Interventions for preventing oral mucositis for patients with cancer receiving treatment. Cochrane Database Syst Rev 2003;3.

Tropical oral infections
Prabhu SR, Wilson DF, Daftary DK, Johnson NW (Eds) Oral Disease in the Tropics. Oxford: Oxford University Press; 1992

Human immunodeficiency virus
Birnbaum W, Hodgson TA, Reichart PA et al. Prognostic significance of HIV-associated oral lesions and their relation to therapy. Oral Dis 2002;8:Suppl 2,110-114.

Herpes virus infections
Naesens L, De Clercq E. Recent developments in herpesvirus therapy. Herpes 2001;8:1,12-16.

Oral candidiasis
Sitheeque MA, Samaranayake LP. Chronic hyperplastic candidosis/candidiasis (candidal leukoplakia). Crit Rev Oral Biol Med 2003;14:4,253-267.

Fidel PL Jr. Immunity to Candida. Oral Dis 2002;8:Suppl 2:69-75.

Chapter 5
White Patches

Aim

The aim of this section is to describe those conditions that present as a white patch on the oral mucosa. Lesions that can predispose to oral cancer will be considered in the next chapter. Some conditions that can present as a white patch on the oral mucosa, such as lichen planus, are described in Chapter 2.

Outcome

After reading this section you should have an understanding of the various disorders of the oral mucosa that present as a white patch, their investigation and management.

Introduction

White patches on the oral mucosa can be broadly divided into those that can be rubbed off and those that cannot. The former comprise three main groups:
- *materia alba* - this is simply the collection of debris, often food, desquamated squames and bacteria
- *Candida* – for example, acute pseudomembranous candidosis
- *dead sloughing mucosa*.

Those white patches that cannot be simply rubbed off are usually a result of either the development of a keratinised layer at a site that is not normally keratinised or thickening of an existing keratinised layer (hyperkeratosis). This produces a change in the texture of the tissue as well as an alteration in the optical properties, giving rise to a characteristic appearance. Although the cause and diagnosis of many of these lesions can be determined from the history or physical appearance, some have similar characteristics and, as a result, can only be differentiated histologically. For this reason, whenever there is any doubt as to the diagnosis of a white lesion, a biopsy is advocated.

Developmental White Lesions

Fordyce granules - these are clusters of creamy white spots, found mainly on the labial and buccal mucosa (Fig 5-1). They are usually asymptomatic,

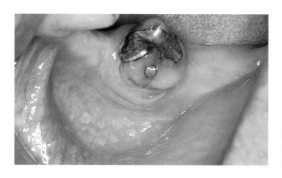

Fig 5-1 Numerous ectopic sebaceous glands in the buccal sulcus (Fordyce spots).

although when noticed by the patient may give rise to cancerophobia. Histologically they represent ectopic sebaceous glands and as such require no more specific treatment than reassurance.

Geographic tongue (erythema migrans) - this common condition of unknown aetiology affects between 2-4% of the population and is characterised by irregular depapilated patches, surrounded by pale, well-demarcated margins (Figs 5-2 and 5-3). The condition predominantly affects the dorsal and lateral margins of the tongue, although similar areas can occasionally be found on other regions of the oral mucosa. The affected areas come and go over a period of days and can present at any age. The condition is usually asymptomatic, although in a few individuals discomfort can follow after eating citrus fruits or spicy foods.

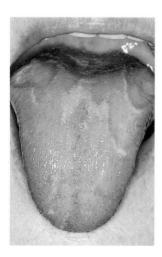

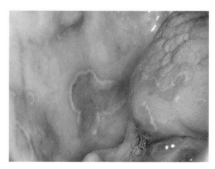

Fig 5-2 (left) Geographic tongue (erythema migrans).

Fig 5-3 (top) Erythema migrans affecting both the tongue and buccal mucosa. By permission of Oxford University Press from "Oral Pathology 4/e" edited by Soames, JV & Southam, JC (2005).

Geographic tongue can usually be diagnosed by its appearance alone, and biopsy is rarely indicated, unless a more sinister lesion is suspected.

The patient should be reassured about the benign nature of the condition. In those with symptoms an underlying haematinic deficiency should be excluded, as for other cases of sore tongue. Unfortunately, symptomatic geographic tongue is often unresponsive to most topical agents, including steroids. Soluble zinc sulphate tablets (45mg zinc) made into a simple mouthwash and used three times daily can provide symptomatic relief for some patients.

Fissured tongue - the appearance of a tongue covered in fissures is not uncommon in clinical practice. Although not a 'white lesion', it frequently accompanies geographic tongue and is entirely benign. Many patients are concerned about this appearance and require frequent reassurance. As in geographic tongue those who complain of symptoms should be investigated to exclude an underlying haematinic deficiency. Usually reassurance alone is all that is needed but simple measures – for example, the use of topical antiseptic agents such chlorhexidine or use of zinc sulphate mouthwashes – may limit discomfort.

White sponge naevus (Fig 5-4) - this is an autosomal dominant condition, with incomplete penetrance, presenting anywhere on the oral mucosa with a shaggy, folded, white appearance. It is usually detected by chance and is one of the few hyperkeratotic conditions of the oral mucosa to occur in young children. It has a distinctive histological appearance and, if there is doubt about the diagnosis, a biopsy is usually confirmatory. No specific treatment is necessary, although genetic counselling should be offered.

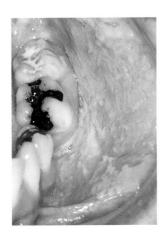

Fig 5-4 White sponge naevus.

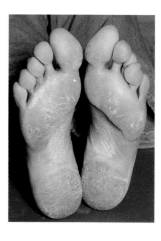

Fig 5-5 Hyperkeratosis of the plantar surface of feet (tylosis).

It is worth noting that white sponge naevus can also affect other mucosal surfaces, including the genitalia and the larynx, and affected patients should be informed of this to prevent what may be unnecessary investigation at a later time.

Tylosis (Fig 5-5) – this is a rare genetic disorder inherited as an autosomal dominant trait characterised by congenital hyperkeratosis of the palms and soles (tylosis). In some patients hyperkeratotic plaques may be present on the oral mucosa. The significance of this condition is its association with the development of oesophageal carcinoma later in life.

Follicular keratosis (Darier's disease) – this uncommon mucocutaneous condition has an autosomal dominant mode of inheritance with variable expressivity. The characteristic skin manifestations includes multiple, heavily keratinised papules that can coalesce, ulcerate and become secondarily infected, producing a foul-smelling mass. Commonly affected sites include the forehead, scalp and ears. Other features include palmar pits and characteristic clefts in the nails. The oral mucosa is involved in approximately 50% of cases, with lesions presenting as whitish, coalescing papules most commonly affecting the hard palate, although they can occur at other sites. In addition, intermittent obstructive sialadenitis of the major salivary glands can occur as a result of changes in the ductal lining, resulting in their narrowing.

Diagnosis of this condition may be made from the family history, although on biopsy the lesions have a characteristic histological appearance. There is no specific treatment required for the oral manifestations of this condition.

Leukoedema - this essentially is a descriptive term where the oral mucosa develops a translucent, milky whiteness, often with a slightly folded texture. It reflects a generalised thickening of the epithelium, is of no specific significance and is not infrequently seen in people with racial pigmentation of the oral mucosa. It also may reflect a reactive change to habits, such as tobacco usage and high alcohol consumption. In these cases the connection should be drawn to patient's attention with advice to modify the habit.

Traumatic Keratoses (Figs 5-6 and 5-7)

The oral mucosa has limited ways to react to an insult and this will depend on the severity, degree and chronicity of the affect. Continual low levels of trauma will result in thickening of the tissue (traumatic hyperkeratosis), and this is most frequently seen on the buccal mucosa or lateral margins of the tongue adjacent to the occlusal plane of the teeth. In most instances the finding requires no specific action, and the characteristic site and appearance provide the diagnosis. However, on the lateral margins of the tongue it may

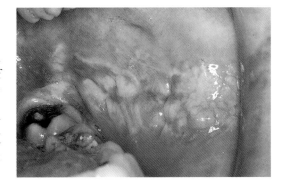

Fig 5-6 Hyperkeratosis adjacent to the occlusal plane of the teeth in a patient who habitually chews his cheek. By permission of Oxford University Press from "Oral Pathology 4/e" edited by Soames, JV & Southam, JC (2005).

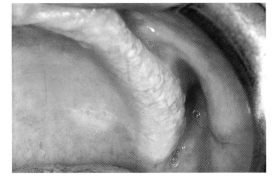

Fig 5-7 Shaggy reactive hyperkeratosis on the upper edentulous alveolar ridge in a patient who prefers not to wear dentures.

mimic other white patches at this site, such as hairy leukoplakia in HIV infection, and as a consequence may require biopsy for confirmation.

In some individuals cheek/tongue/lip chewing is a habitual problem and can result in quite dramatic damage and hyperkeratosis to the affected sites. Such a habit can be difficult to control but in those who request treatment smoothing of sharp cusps, or the provision of a soft vinyl blow-down occlusal coverage splint for wear during times of the habit activity, may be helpful. The condition has no other serious connotations.

Similar reactive hyperkeratosis can occur in an edentulous area of the alveolar ridge, which becomes used as a surrogate tooth surface. The appearance characteristically is of a shaggy keratosis limited to the affected area, and as a consequence its diagnosis is usually made on clinical grounds, although as with other white lesions if there is any doubt a biopsy will be confirmatory.

Chemical trauma - the application of caustic chemicals to the oral mucosa will result in tissue death and resulting sloughing of the superficial layers, which, when scrapped away, reveal an ulcerated and often bleeding surface. Classically this condition is associated with aspirin placed on the oral mucosa and allowed to dissolve – for example, in the treatment of toothache (Fig 5-8). In most cases the history is all that is required to make the diagnosis and treatment is symptomatic, with the use of antiseptic mouthwashes such as chlorhexidine.

Thermal trauma - burns can occur anywhere on the oral mucosa, most frequently the anterior palate, as a result of eating food that is too hot, particularly any that is likely to stick, such as molten cheese. The treatment for this would be symptomatic, as indicated in previous sections.

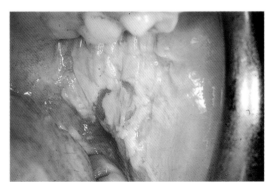

Fig 5-8 Dead sloughing epithelium on the buccal mucosa as a result of using an aspirin topically (aspirin burn).

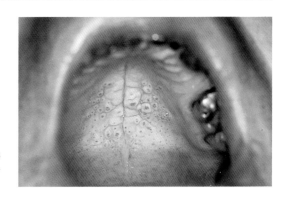

Fig 5-9 Nicotinic stomatitis in a patient who is a long-term pipe smoker.

Regular heavy smokers not infrequently develop hyperkeratotic changes on their oral mucosa as a response to both the chemical and thermal irritation from their smoking habit (Fig 5-9). This condition is most frequently seen on the palate (nicotinic stomatitis) where it can result in a blockage of the minor salivary ducts, which become inflamed, giving a characteristic clinical appearance. Although smoking-related, this condition is considered benign but obviously indicates a reaction about which the patient should be informed. The problem will usually gradually resolve on cessation of the habit.

Conclusions

- White patches can be fixed or removable – check first.
- Many hyperkeratotic lesions can appear very similar.
- History and clinical examination are important in making the differential diagnosis.
- If there is any doubt about the diagnosis a biopsy is essential.

Further Reading

Soames JV, Southam JC. Oral Pathology 4th ed. Oxford: Oxford Medical Publicatons, 2005.

Chapter 6

Oral Cancer and Premalignant Lesions

Aim

This chapter describes the diagnosis and management of oral cancer.

Outcome

After reading this chapter you should have an understanding of the management of oral cancer and be familiar with those conditions that are premalignant.

Introduction

Squamous cell carcinoma arising from the surface epithelium accounts for approximately 90% of all malignant disease affecting the mouth. On a global basis it is the sixth most common cancer to affect humankind. There are marked variations, with the highest incidence in the developing countries, where it is up to the third most common malignancy. In the West it accounts for approximately 4.2% of all cancers, although there are some regional variations, such as a relatively high level in the Bas-Rhin region of France. These variations probably reflect underlying aetiological factors. There is a slightly lower incidence in the US, where it accounts for 2% of all cancers. In the UK there are approximately 3,500 new cases per annum, with a five-year survival rate of around 50%. The survival rate of oral cancer is lower than for many other malignancies, which often have a higher public profile and awareness.

In addition to being the primary site for a malignancy to arise the mouth can also be an area where metastatic disease appears (Fig 6-1).

Risk Factors

Although oral cancer can arise in a variety of 'pre-cancerous conditions', the majority of cases appear to arise *de novo* in clinically normal tissue. The aetiology is almost certainly multi-factorial, but there are a number of apparent risk factors:

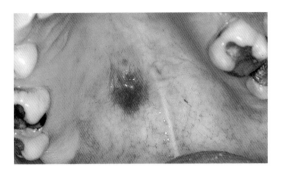

Fig 6-1 Exopytic, highly vascular lesion on palate, which suddenly appeared in a patient with a history of renal carcinoma. This lesion transpired to be a metastasis.

Age – the prevalence of oral cancer increases with age. In the UK 90% of patients are over 40, although alarmingly there is a rising incidence in those under 35 years old, which may reflect changes in social habits.

Tobacco – tobacco usage in all its forms, whether smoked or chewed, increases the risk of developing oral cancer. There is a smoking history in over 60% of affected patients and in 80% of those where the disease is in the floor of the mouth.

Alcohol – consumption of alcohol above the recommended safe drinking limits (21 units for a male and 14 units for a female) is found in 24% of all patients with oral cancer and in 41% of those whose disease is in the floor of mouth. The combination of heavy tobacco usage and alcohol consumption appears to operate in a multiplicative (synergistic) fashion, producing a 40 times increased risk over those who do not smoke and stay within safe drinking limits.

Areca (Betel nut) – the use of areca nut often in combination with tobacco and other constituents (paan-quid-gutkha) placed in the buccal sulcus and left for considerable periods of time is a relatively common habit among various Asian communities. It is associated with an increased risk of developing squamous cell carcinoma in the mouth.

All the above factors depend, to some degree, on the frequency and duration of use by having a direct local effect. In the case of alcohol and tobacco there may be additional systemic effects.

Other Possible Risk Factors

Other risk factors for oral malignancy include:
- dietary deficiencies, particularly of vitamins A, C and E and iron, and trace elements such as selenium and zinc
- viral infections – for example, certain types of human papilloma viruses (HPVs)
- candidal infection
- excessive exposure to sunlight or UV radiation (for lip cancer)
- immune deficiency disease or immunosuppression
- possible familial or genetic predisposition
- environmental pollutants
- mutation of p53 cancer suppression gene – possibly as a result of smoking or HPV infection
- chronic oral sepsis – this factor may be the result of local irritation to adjacent tissues but also reflects a general poor health awareness.

Clinical Features

Squamous cell cancer of the mouth can present in many ways and can occur at any site, with the most frequent being floor of mouth and ventral/lateral margins of tongue (Fig 6-2). The following clinical signs should be regarded with great suspicion:
- any ulcer of the mucosa that fails to heal within two to three weeks
- any area of firmness (induration) of the oral tissue
- fungation/growth of the tissues to produce an elevated, cauliflower surface or lump
- fixation of any lesion to underlying tissues with loss of normal mobility
- failure to heal of a tooth socket, or any other wound
- tooth mobility with no apparent cause
- pain/paraesthesia with no apparent cause

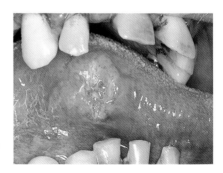

Fig 6-2 Squamous cell carcinoma on lateral margin of tongue.

- difficulty in swallowing (dysphagia) for which no other diagnosis can be made
- white/red patches of the mucosa – these are commonly considered as potentially malignant lesions, but occasionally may represent an early-phase squamous cell carcinoma
- lymphadenopathy – any large, particularly asymptomatic lymph node in the submental, submandibular and cervical chain area should be regarded with suspicion, and if persistent referred for either surgical removal or fine-needle aspiration cytology.

It should be emphasised, however, that the majority of early oral carcinomas are often entirely asymptomatic.

Management

Squamous cell carcinoma is probably the most life-threatening disorder to affect the mouth and the dental practitioner is in a key position to advise on prevention, its early recognition and appropriate referral for treatment.

As a routine all health care workers should be prepared to give advice regarding known risk factors, in particular smoking and alcohol consumption. A thorough oral examination should always be undertaken and any suspicious lesions noted. Biopsy is obligatory to confirm the diagnosis. If a malignancy is suspected it is best to refer to the appropriate specialist as a matter of urgency for a biopsy. If it is decided to keep a lesion under review this should be within two to three weeks, allowing most inflammatory (traumatic) lesions to settle.

Routine screening of patients for oral cancer using a variety of techniques, including tolonium chloride dye or brush cytology of suspected lesions (or following areas highlighted by tolonium chloride) has been advocated on a regular basis for high-risk groups. However, the efficacy of such procedures remains somewhat controversial.

Biopsy

As mentioned above where a malignant/potentially malignant lesion is considered in general practice the biopsy would probably be better undertaken by the person who is going to provide the definitive treatment, as it allows them to relate the site of biopsy to the planning of further treatment. This will also take into account the extent of the lesion and its possible spread (staging) as indicated clinically or by various imaging modalities such as com-

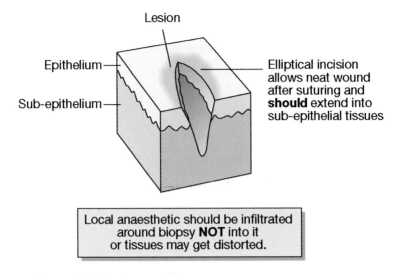

Lesion

Epithelium

Sub-epithelium

Elliptical incision allows neat wound after suturing and **should** extend into sub-epithelial tissues

Local anaesthetic should be infiltrated around biopsy **NOT** into it or tissues may get distorted.

Fig 6-3 Taking an incisional mucosal biopsy.

puted tomography (CT) or magnetic resonance imaging (MRI). The process of taking a mucosal biopsy under local anaesthesia can be found in any standard textbook on oral surgery. When taken to assess the possibility of malignant disease or dysplasia it is essential that a representative site be selected and an adequate sample size taken (Fig 6-3). This may involve taking samples from two or more sites to ensure a representative indication of what is happening to the tissues. More recently disposable punch biopsies have been advocated. These are simple to use, with the 4 or 6mm size being adequate for most oral lesions, and the wound may not require suturing after the procedure. If this technique is used then selection of a representative site(s) is imperative.

Treatment
At present oral cancer is treated primarily by surgery. The lesion is excised along with a reasonable margin of apparently healthy tissue. The local regional lymph nodes may also be removed at the same time and the deficit repaired using a variety of reconstructive techniques, details of which can be found in texts on maxillofacial surgery (see further reading). Radiotherapy is often used as an adjunct to surgery or as the main treatment modality for those cases that are unsuitable for surgery. To-date chemotherapy has proved to be relatively ineffective in the management of oral cancer. In general terms, the more anterior in the mouth the lesion is the better the prognosis. The

most important factor in the eventual outcome, however, is its stage at presentation.

Lifestyle Counselling

The opportunity to talk to patients on a one-to-one basis about lifestyle issues is now regarded as an important role for health care workers, including those in the dental team. Advice about smoking cessation or reducing alcohol consumption is best done on a one-to-one basis, in a way that leaves the patient feeling in control and able to stop the conversation if it gets too uncomfortable.

Where lifestyle issues have been discussed with patients these should be recorded in their records, as at a subsequent visit the issue can be raised again. This emphasises the importance placed on the advice given.

Where a practitioner is concerned regarding the appearance of an oral lesion, this should be conveyed to the patient as tactfully as possible, using simple language such as 'there appears to be a red/white patch in your mouth and I am not sure what it is'. This could be followed up with something along the lines of 'I would like to get a colleague who sees more of these sorts of things than myself to have a look', and an arrangement to see the appropriate specialist made, preferably while the patient is still present, so that the appointment can be given directly. A formal referral letter should also be sent, indicating the background and reasons for the concern and noting what action has been taken to date. A record of the patient's medical history, alcohol and tobacco habits as well as contact details and those of the general medical practitioner should also be included.

Epithelial Dysplasia

This is a histological description indicating an alteration in the tissue architecture, as well as the presence of abnormal cells or cell division. The pathologist usually indicates the degree as mild, moderate or severe, depending on how far up the epithelium these changes are noted. The degree of dysplasia is widely believed to be an indicator of the likelihood of a malignant transformation, although there is actually little evidence to support this. In addition it is now recognised that the presence of dysplasia does not necessarily mean that the lesion is committed to eventual malignant transformation. In some instances, particularly if factors such as smoking are removed, areas of mild or moderate dysplasia can revert back to normal.

A lesion in which dysplastic features extend the full thickness of the epithelium, but where the basement membrane remains intact, are termed 'carcinoma in situ' and are best regarded and managed as an early carcinoma.

Potentially Malignant Lesions

A lesion can be regarded as potentially malignant when it is associated with a significantly increased risk of developing into a carcinoma. Pre-cancerous lesions are usually well demarcated, but the clinical signs are often less obvious than those for an established cancer. The diagnosis, referral, management and follow-up of patients with these lesions, however, is important. Such lesions are described below.

Leukoplakia (Figs 6-4 to 6-7)
This is defined as a white patch or plaque on the oral mucosa that cannot be rubbed off and cannot be characterised clinically or histologically as any other disease.

Oral leukoplakia may have no obvious cause (idiopathic) or be associated with any of the risk factors outlined for oral carcinoma.

There is some debate as to what proportion of these lesions undergo malignant change, but it has been estimated that between 2-6% undergo malignant transformation over a 10-year period. Those on the floor of mouth/ventral surface of tongue may be at greater risk, with some studies suggesting that 25% will undergo malignant transformation.

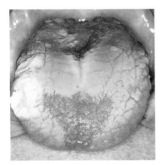

Fig 6-4 Leukoplakia affecting the dorsum of tongue. Note the thickened area on the right lateral margin, which would be the site of most concern and warrant biopsy.

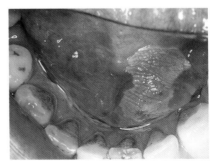

Fig 6-5 Hyperkeratosis (leukoplakia) on the floor of mouth in a smoker.

79

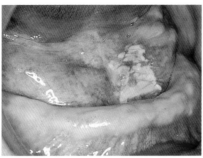

Fig 6-6 Hyperkeratotic lesion on floor of mouth with associated red areas. This lesion on biopsy transpired to be an early squamous cell carcinoma.

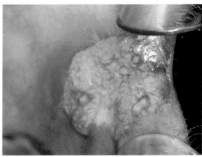

Fig 6-7 Speckled leukoplakia of the oral commissure. On biopsy this dysplastic lesion was associated with candida.

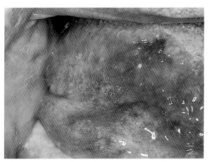

Fig 6-8 Erythroplakia on lateral margin of tongue.

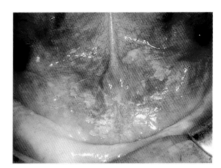

Fig 6-9 Erythroplakia on floor of mouth.

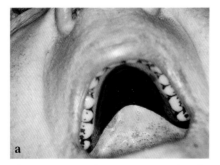

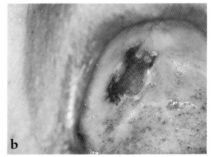

Fig 6-10 Irregular, asymptomatic, ulcerated lesion on palate covered by a heavily tar-stained upper denture (a) in a long-term heavy pipe smoker. On biopsy the lesion transpired to be a squamous cell carcinoma(b).

Clinical Appearance

Homogenous Leukoplakia

This appears as a uniform white plaque anywhere in the mouth. The surface may be smooth or cracked in appearance.

Non-Homogenous Leukoplakia

This can have either a warty, hyperplastic or nodular surface and is not infrequently associated with *Candida albicans* infection.

Speckled Leukoplakia

This has combined red and white elements in the plaque and has an irregular surface texture. The appearance of this lesion is often associated with severe dysplasia. It may even be an early carcinoma and, as a consequence, warrants urgent investigation and management.

Erythroplakia (Figs 6–8 and 6–9)

This is defined as a bright red velvet plaque on the oral mucosa that cannot be characterised clinically or pathologically as being due to any other condition.

Common sites for erythroplakia are the buccal mucosa, soft palate and lateral tongue. Generally erythroplakia has a higher malignant potential than leukoplakia. Biopsy frequently shows changes ranging from mild dysplasia to early invasive squamous cell carcinoma. As a consequence the finding of an unusual red patch on the oral mucosa should be regarded with high suspicion and managed accordingly.

Management

Biopsy to assess the degree of dysplasia is essential for all cases of leukoplakia or erythroplakia. Where this is found to be minimal the lesion could be excised if relatively small, removed using laser ablation or regularly monitored. There is some evidence that the use of vitamin A analogues (retinoids) can be effective in cases of leukoplakia, although recurrence may occur once treatment is stopped. Obviously where a causative factor can be identified – for example, smoking – advice regarding habit cessation should be given. In all cases careful follow-up is advised.

Other Potentially Premalignant Conditions

Chronic Iron Deficiency Anaemia

Paterson-Kelly (Plummer-Vinson) syndrome is a combination of iron deficiency anaemia with dysphagia and glossitis. Mucosal atrophy is a common feature of chronic iron deficiency and appears to predispose the affected tissues to malignant transformation.

Erosive Lichen Planus

This is described in Chapter 2.

Oral Submucous Fibrosis

This condition presents as a loss of elasticity of the mucosa as a result of the development of fibrous bands in the submucosa, causing limitation of opening of the mouth. The tongue shows loss of papillae, firmness and a lack of mobility. A burning sensation in the mouth or throat may be an early symptom. The condition is most common in Asian communities and possibly reflects a reaction to use of areca nut or significant quantities of chillies in the diet.

The management of this condition is prevention with lifestyle counselling and also in careful monitoring for changes. A biopsy is essential to assess the degree of underlying epithelial dysplasia.

Lupus Erythematosis

This is described in Chapter 2.

Tertiary Syphilis

This condition is now rare in the UK, as syphilis is usually diagnosed and treated at an earlier stage. The tertiary phase frequently affects the tongue (syphilitic glossitis) and presents as a combination of keratotic plaques and epithelial atrophy. The condition is usually diagnosed by a combination of biopsy and serological markers for syphilis. There is some controversy over this condition, as many affected patients may have used arsenic-containing products in the past. These were frequently used in the treatment of syphilis and can lead to problems with malignancy, particularly of the mucous membranes and skin, later in life.

Actinic Keratosis

This condition is most frequently seen on exposed skin and the lower lip. It is caused by long-term exposure to ultraviolent light and is consequently most likely seen in people who spend substantial amounts of time out of doors, such as farmers or seamen, and in those who have spent considerable time in hot climates. The condition is characterised by combinations of erosion and white or brown crusting.

Management of this condition usually involves patient education about further exposure to strong sunlight and surgical removal of suspicious areas. Regular follow-up is also advisable.

Conclusions

- All health care workers should be prepared to council about known risk factors for oral cancer, such as smoking and excessive alcohol consumption.
- Squamous cell carcinoma is the commonest malignancy to affect the oral mucosa.
- Surviving oral cancer depends on its early detection.
- The degree of epithelial dysplasia may determine the chance of malignant transformation.

Further Reading

Pedlar J, Frame JW. Oral and Maxillofacial Surgery. London: Churchill Livingstone, 2001 (pp125-142).

Scully C, Flint SR, Porter SR. Oral Diseases. London: Martin Dunitz, 1996.

Soames JV, Southam JC. Oral Pathology 4th ed. Oxford: Oxford Medical Publications 2005.

Chapter 7
Oral Pigmentation

Aim

The aim of this section is to describe the various disorders that can give rise to pigmentation of the oral mucosa.

Outcome

After reading this chapter you should have an understanding of the various conditions that can produce pigmentation of the oral mucosa, their significance, investigation and management.

Introduction

Oral pigmentation can occur as a result of deposition of exogenous pigmented substances into or on the surface of the mucosa. Alternatively it may occur as a result of deposition into the tissues of pigments produced by the body (endogenous). These latter pigments are usually melanin but may also include blood pigments such as haemosiderin.

Superficial Staining
This may be caused by a variety of food colourings, medicaments or tobacco products, and its only significance is as an indicator of the usage of such products.

Black Hairy Tongue (Fig 7-1)
This condition arises as a result of elongation of the filiform papillae and subsequent discoloration from chromogenic bacteria. The exact cause is unknown, although there is a suggestion that it may be more common in smokers and in full-denture wearers. There is no particular significance to this condition, although its appearance often concerns patients. Treatment usually involves improvement of oral hygiene, including gently scraping the surface of the tongue with either a custom-made tongue scraper or soft toothbrush.

Amalgam Tattoo (Figs 7-2 and 7-3)
This relatively common lesion usually presents as an asymptomatic

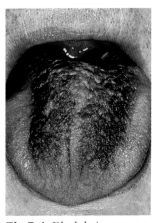

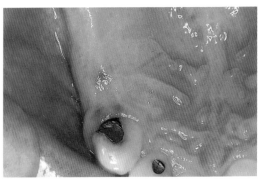

Fig 7-2 Purplish blue discoloration of the upper alveolar ridge due to implanted amalgam (amalgam tattoo).

Fig 7-1 Black hairy tongue.

blue/black pigmented area and is often a chance finding during routine oral examination. It arises as a result of amalgam debris being implanted into the soft tissues. This subsequently breaks down releasing silver salts, which produce the staining. As a consequence, if observed over a period of time these lesions may appear to enlarge and undergo a degree of colour change. There is no specific significance to this condition, apart from its diagnosis, which could either be done by an intra-oral radiograph demonstrating the amalgam debris within the tissues, or biopsy.

Foreign Material
A variety of foreign substances implanted into the tissues can give rise to staining. These include graphite from pencils and deliberate tattooing. There is no specific significance to these lesions apart from their diagnosis, which

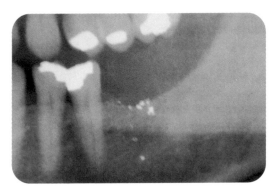

Fig 7-3 A radiograph demonstrating the presence of amalgram debris within the tissue in a patient with an amalgam tattoo.

may be either self-evident or through the history, although where there is doubt a biopsy will be confirmatory.

Heavy Metal Salts

Deposits of heavy metals that have been ingested, such as lead or bismuth, can be precipitated, usually as sulphides along the gingival margin producing a characteristic blue line. The significance of this is the effect on general health rather than specifically to the oral tissues.

Melanin Pigmentation

Melanin is secreted by dendritic cells (melanocytes) positioned along the basal layer of the epithelium. The pigment can be expressed either as a result of an acquired cause or be developmental.

Developmental Causes

Racial Pigmentation

Races with dark skin frequently exhibit patches of melanin pigment on their oral mucosa that are of no specific consequence.

Pigmented Naevi

Melanotic naevi are relatively common on the skin, as a result of collections of melanocytes developing usually at the dermo/epidermal junction, or in the dermis. A range of such naevi are recognisable histologically, such as junctional, compound or intradermal and their significance is really as a potential for the development of malignant melanoma. Although pigmented naevi can occur in the oral tissues, they are extremely rare, and the treatment usually involves excision.

Peutz-Jegher Syndrome

This inherited syndrome is characterised by mucocutaneous melanotic macules, most commonly circumoral, and intestinal polyps. The latter most frequently occur in the small intestine, where they can lead to intussusception. The polyps rarely undergo malignant change, unlike those in polyposis coli (see Gardner's syndrome, see page 46).

The diagnosis of Peutz-Jegher syndrome is clinical, but in view of the intestinal polyps patients should be followed up by a gastroenterologist.

Acquired Causes

In the oral mucosa most melanocytes could be considered as dormant but

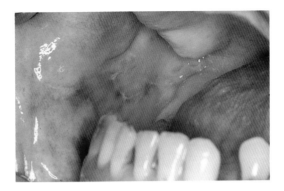

Fig 7-4 Melanin pigmentation associated with lichen planus. Such pigmentation may remain for some time after the original lesion has settled.

can be stimulated as a result of local or systemic factors. Local factors include chronic inflammation, and as a consequence pigmentation can be seen accompanying conditions such as oral lichen planus or leukoplakia (Fig 7-4).

Oral Focal Melanosis (Figs 7-5 and 7-6)

This asymptomatic condition usually presents as either multiple or solitary patches of melanin pigmentation around the oral mucosa. In many cases the problem is idiopathic and may need to be differentiated from Addison's disease (see below). However, a similar picture can also occasionally be seen in smokers where it may be the result of stimulation of melanocytes as a result of irritation from the combination of heat and chemicals in tobacco smoke. A variation of this condition is the solitary melanotic macule that occurs characteristically on the lower lip. There is no specific significance to these conditions apart from their diagnosis. In patients who smoke the implication of this

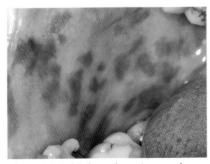

Fig 7-5 Multiple melanotic macules on the buccal mucosa in a patient with oral focal melanosis.

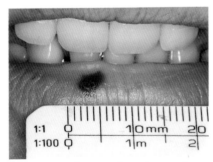

Fig 7-6 A solitary melanotic macule on the lower lip.

factor as an indicator of mucosal reaction needs to be made, although the condition can last for some considerable time once the habit is stopped.

Solitary melanotic macules of the lower lip frequently cause cosmetic problems and as a result should either be surgically removed or treated using cryotherapy.

Addison's Disease
Addison's disease occurs as a result of adrenocortical damage and resultant hypofunction following autoimmune damage, tuberculosis or carcinomatosis. It results in hypotension and, with a loss of the negative feedback control to the anterior pituitary, an over-production of adrenocorticotrophic hormone (ACTH). This excess of ACTH stimulates the melanocytes, producing a generalised hyperpigmentation of the skin and mucosae. It particularly affects skin flexures, the genitalia and sites of trauma.

Diagnosis
Addison's disease may need to be differentiated from other causes of diffuse oral hyperpigmentation, such as oral focal melanosis and drug-induced pigmentation. Generally the adrenal hypofunction is determined by:
- reduced blood pressure
- reduced plasma cortisol levels
- low or no response to synthetic ACTH stimulation (Synacthen test).

Management
Addison's disease is managed using replacement corticosteroid therapy.

Drug-Induced Hyperpigmentation
Various drugs can cause pigmentation, although the mechanisms of how this occurs are poorly understood. Drugs commonly implicated include:
- antimalarials
- busulphan
- cisplatin
- phenothiazines
- zidovudine
- oral contraceptives.

The diagnosis of this problem is usually from the history of drug usage and there is no specific significance to the condition.

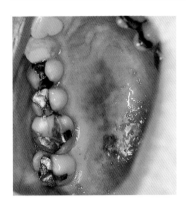

Fig 7-7 An early malignant melanoma on the hard palate. Note the irregular margins and variable degree of pigmentation within the lesion.

Malignant Melanoma (Fig 7-7)

Although malignant melanoma is not an uncommon neoplasm of the skin it is fortunately rare in the oral cavity, where the most likely site for its development is in the palate.

Clinical Features

Malignant melanoma may present as a solitary asymptomatic, brown or black macule. The depth of pigmentation may vary throughout the lesion and the margin may be irregular. Growth can either be exophytic, producing a lump, or by superficial spread through the mucosa, producing an increasing area of pigmentation. Metastatic spread from melanomas can be quite rapid and occur at a relatively early stage. As a consequence it is not unknown for a patient to present as a result of metastatic disease, such as enlarged lymph nodes or to the lungs or liver before the primary lesion is identified.

Diagnosis

Malignant melanomas are diagnosed by biopsy and the prognosis to some degree is determined by the depth of invasion seen.

Treatment

Malignant melanomas are best treated by total surgical removal, although in a number of cases the presentation may be quite late and the prognosis is often poor. Recent developments in the use of chemo- and immunotherapy may improve the outlook.

Conclusions

• Pigmented lesions in the oral mucosa are not uncommon.

- Most melanotic oral mucosal lesions are either idiopathic or due to local irritation.
- Underlying systemic causes should be considered, especially if there are other medical symptoms or signs present.
- Oral pigmentation can be due to certain medications.
- Melanotic naevi and malignant melanoma are rare in the mouth.

Further Reading

Scully C, Flint SR. Oral Diseases. London: Martin Dunitz, 1996.

Soames JV, Southam JC. Oral Pathology 4th ed. Oxford: Oxford Medical Publications, 2005.

Chapter 8
Disorders of Salivary Glands and Salivation

Aim

The aim of this chapter is to describe the various disorders that can affect the salivary glands and salivation.

Outcome

After reading this chapter you should have an understanding of the various disorders that can affect the salivary glands and salivation, their investigation and management.

Introduction

Disorders of salivary glands and salivation are relatively common and for the purpose of this chapter are classified into the following categories:
• salivary flow disturbance
• salivary gland infections
• salivary gland swellings.

Salivary Flow Disturbance

The lining of the mouth is kept moist by saliva, a complex fluid that helps keep it in a healthy state. The body produces approximately 1.5 litres of saliva per day with resting flow rates undergoing a circadian rhythm fluctuation that is constant from day to day. The resting flow rate is at its lowest during the night. Thus patients with low levels of saliva experience their worst symptoms during this time. Salivary flow can be stimulated by chewing or by the thought or smell of food. It can be diminished by emotions such as anxiety.

Sources of Saliva

Full saliva is produced by the salivary glands, both major and minor. The major salivary glands are the paired parotid, submandibular and sublingual glands. Congenital absence of one or more of these glands can occur but is rare. The minor salivary glands are numerous and scattered around the mouth but predominantly around the lips and the junction of the hard and soft palate.

Composition and Functions of Saliva

Analysis of the components of saliva presents many difficulties. Its composition varies from person to person and at different times in one individual. The relative amounts of each component differ depending on the relative contribution from each source. This, in turn, is dependent on the stimulus and circumstances at the time. In general, the parotids produce watery or serous saliva while the sublingual and minor glands produce thicker and more viscous (mucous) saliva. The submandibular glands produce combinations of both. Details of the exact composition of saliva are outwith the scope of this book and the reader is recommended to seek further details in a standard text on oral biology. The chief functions of saliva are:
• mucosal protection – lubrication and tissue repair
• microbial control – bacteria, fungi and some viruses
• alimentation – gustation, bolus formation and translocation
• digestion – especially in the initiation of complex carbohydrate breakdown
• remineralisation of teeth – through presence of calcium and phosphate
• buffering – pH maintenance.

It can be seen from the above list that changes in either the quantity or composition of saliva can have a significant effect on the health of the oral tissues.

Measurement of Salivary Flow (Sialometry)

Measurement of salivary flow rates may be useful in assessing the severity of disease in the glands. Full saliva can be collected by allowing it to drain into a collecting cup over a period of time, usually over a 15-minute period (normal >1.5ml), ensuring that no swallowing occurs. The difficulty with the method is preventing mechanical stimulation. In addition, drawing attention to salivation may in itself cause stimulation. It is possible to measure stimulated salivary flow by getting the patient to chew on an inert substance, such as gum or a rubber band, then getting them to spit into a pot again over a period of time, usually five minutes, then measuring or weighing the quantity produced. To measure the flow rate of individual major glands, cannulation of the salivary duct or the use of small collecting chambers that fit over the duct opening may be used.

'The Dry Mouth' (Xerostomia)

The complaint of having a dry mouth is common and can arise from either a change in sensation or reduction in the amount of saliva produced (Fig 8-1). As with all conditions, it is essential to take a thorough history of the complaint and any associated features. The history should include details of a patient's smoking habits and alcohol consumption. The former can have a drying effect on oral tissues and the latter may cause dehydration. Patients with a reduced quantity of saliva will almost invariably indicate that their symptoms are worse at night. They complain of waking frequently and having to have sips of water to try and relubricate their oral tissues. In addition to their dryness they may also indicate problems with swallowing. They may have adapted their diet accordingly, avoiding dry foods and having to drink fluid in order to swallow. They may also state that food has lost its taste. It is often these latter features that patients find most distressing.

Clinical examination of a patient with dry mouth follows the same pattern as for those with other conditions, although certain signs may be apparent. On giving their history it may be noticed that the speech has a clicking quality as a result of the tongue sticking to the palatal mucosa. The oral tissues will appear dry and somewhat atrophic, this being most apparent on the tongue, which frequently becomes depapilated with a lobulated surface.

In severe cases of dry mouth only scant (or no) saliva will be expressible from the main ducts. This can sometimes happen in the otherwise healthy patient as a result of anxiety, but simple stimulation through the application of a drop of lemon juice to the mouth should differentiate a temporary from a more permanent problem.

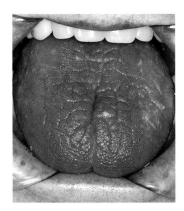

Fig 8-1 Severe xerostomia. Note how the lingual mucosa has become atrophic and fissured. This patient has Sjögren's syndrome

Causes for Dry Mouth

A number of conditions can cause xerostomia. These are discussed below.

Sjögren's Syndrome (Figs 8-1 and 8-2)

The combination of dryness of the eyes (xerophthalmia) and mouth (xerostomia) due to an autoimmune, chronic inflammatory damage to the lacrimal and salivary glands was first described by Sjögren in the 1930s. When these two features appear alone the condition is referred to as primary Sjögren's syndrome, when associated with various connective tissue disorders - such as rheumatoid arthritis, systemic lupus erythematosis, systemic sclerosis, CREST syndrome and primary biliary cirrhosis - it is known as secondary Sjögren's syndrome. It is estimated that around 15% of patients with rheumatoid arthritis will also have symptoms of dry eyes and dry mouth.

Like with many other autoimmune conditions there is a tendency for females to be affected more than males. In some instances the condition is familial. Its onset is insidious and consequently tends to present over the age of 30.

Although regarded as principally involving the eyes and mouth, the condition can also be associated with a variety of other effects, such as a dry vagina, irritable bowel-type symptoms and other manifestations. Patients (and occasionally their medical advisers) may be unaware of the connection. The term Sicca syndrome was previously used as an alternative name for primary Sjögren's syndrome, although more recently it has been suggested that this term be used only for those who, despite their symptoms, have a negative labial gland biopsy (see below).

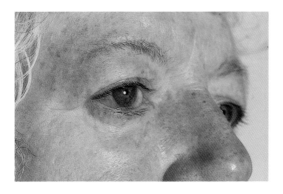

Fig 8-2 Conjunctivitis as a result of dry eyes (xerophthalmia) in a patient with Sjögren's syndrome. By permission of Oxford University Press from "Oral Pathology 4/e" edited by Soames, JV & Southam, JC (2005).

Pathogensis

Viral, genetic and immune factors are thought to be involved in the pathogensis of Sjögren's syndrome. Ro and La extractable antinuclear antibodies (ENA) are found in approximately 80% and 50% respectively of cases, particularly with primary Sjögren's syndrome.

Histologically the salivary glands are infiltrated by lymphocytes, resulting in acinar destruction with fibrosis and myoepithelial cell proliferation, which may form 'islands' and ductal damage. The identification of foci of lymphocytes forms the basis of diagnosis from the labial gland biopsy (see below). The lymphocyte infiltration may become gross, resulting in gland enlargement forming a pseudolymphoma. In some cases a malignant B-cell lymphoma may develop, with resultant rapid enlargement of the affected gland.

Diagnosis

A number of diagnostic tests may be used. These include:

- Labial gland biopsy – regarded as the 'gold standard' diagnostic test for Sjögren's syndrome. Between five to seven minor labial glands are removed through a vertical incision in the lower lip adjacent to the canine. Histological confirmation involves finding several foci of lymphocytic infiltration.
- Salivary flow measures (sialometry) – these tests are somewhat unreliable and time-consuming to perform and consequently are not always undertaken routinely. They can be useful, however, in reassuring patients who have otherwise normal flow levels.
- Tear secretion (Schirmer test) – placement of strip of filter paper under the lower eyelid and left with the eyes closed for five minutes. Wetting of the filter paper 5mm or less after this period is considered positive.
- Autoantibodies – autoantibodies associated with the various connective tissue disorders should be investigated, including rheumatoid factor, antinuclear factor and antimitrochondrial antibodies. Specific ENA antibodies, such as anti Ro and La, are present in a significant proportion of patients with Sjögren's syndrome.
- Nuclear medicine studies – reduced uptake of technetium by salivary glands. This investigation is relatively non-specific but does give an overview of gland activity.
- Sialography – classically shows a 'snow storm' or 'cherry blossom' appearance due to sialectasia (Fig 8-3).

An oral rinse or mucosal smear should be taken to investigate the presence of Candida if there is any soreness.

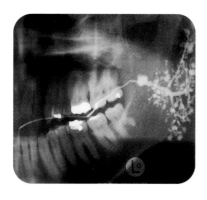

Fig 8-3 Punctate and globular sialectasia demonstrated on left parotid sialogram in a patient with Sjögren's syndrome.

Management

Currently it is not possible to control the underlying autoimmune disease in Sjögren's syndrome. Patients do require careful follow-up, however, because of the implications of having a dry mouth. Problems include increased caries rate, particularly of the incisal edges and smooth surfaces, increased susceptibility to periodontal disease and increased liability to oral infections, particularly candidiasis. In addition the possibility of development of lymphoma needs to be considered. Patients who have significant problems from their dry eyes should be advised to see an ophthalmologist because of the risk of conjunctivitis, corneal damage and resultant blindness. Dry eyes are usually managed with artificial tears (hypomellose eye drops) or on occasions by the temporary or permanent obliteration of the tear duct, reducing the drainage of the small quantity of tears that may be secreted.

Management of Oral Problems

It is wise to advise patients to avoid things that may exacerbate their xerostomia – for example, drugs with a sympathomimetic effect, alcohol, smoking and dry foods such as biscuits.

Artificial Salivary Substitutes and Stimulants

A whole range of artificial saliva preparations is available, mostly based on either carboxymethylcellulose (for example, Glandosane) or mucin (for example, Saliva Orthana). The former products may have a low pH that could damage teeth and should be avoided in dentate patients. Preferably products with a more neutral pH containing fluoride should be selected. Recently oral hygiene products (toothpaste and mouthwash) have been developed to use in conjunction with saliva replacement gels. These contain enzyme systems that protect the oral environment as well as providing lubrication.

Many patients find the various saliva substitutes unhelpful and often resort to more simple measures, such as frequent sipping of water or even rinsing the mouth with olive oil. There have been some reports in the literature of a positive effect on saliva production using acupuncture.

Chewing gum – the act of chewing stimulates saliva. Varieties containing sugar should be avoided. Specialist gums that also contain lubricant and enzymes are available for patients with dry mouth.

Diabetic sweets and pastilles – these may be used to stimulate salivary flow without increasing caries.

Cholinergic drugs – these drugs, such as pilocarpine, stimulate salivation. This can be effective but unfortunately is frequently associated with side-effects such as bradycardia, sweating and the urge to urinate.

Vaseline – lips should be protected by vaseline or some other greasy preparation.

Dental Caries and Periodontal Disease
With the loss of the protective saliva dental disease can become rampant – thus regular review in conjunction with meticulous oral hygiene is essential. Patients should be advised to control intake of fermentable carbohydrates, and in severe cases daily use of fluoride mouthwashes is recommended.

Candidiasis
Candidiasis is a common complication of having a dry mouth and may present with soreness or a burning sensation of the oral tissues. It should be treated accordingly with either a topical antifungal, such as miconazole gel, or systemic antifungal, such as fluconazole. In the denture-wearing patient it is essential to ensure good denture hygiene. In particular patients should be discouraged from wearing dentures at night and advised to store them in a solution of either chlorhexidine or sodium hypochlorite.

Bacterial Sialadenitis
Occasionally an ascending bacterial sialadenitis, most frequently affecting the parotids, can arise as a complication of dry mouth. This should be treated promptly, using an antibiotic such as flucloxacillin.

Other Causes of Dry Mouth
Other causes of xerostomia include:

- Drugs – probably the most common cause (Table 8-1) and often due to sympathomimetic side-effects. In addition, dry mouth can also occur with various self-prescribed preparations, such as decongestant cold remedies.
- Radiotherapy to the head and neck involving salivary glands – this will produce either a temporary or permanent reduction in salivary flow, as salivary tissue is radiosensitive. Some improvement in function may occur with time and, providing there are no contraindications, salivary stimulating agents, such as pilocarpine, may be beneficial.
- Dehydration.
- Diabetes mellitus – uncontrolled diabetic patients may develop a dry mouth as a result of dehydration. The possibility of diabetes needs to be considered in patients who in addition to presenting with a dry mouth complain of thirst and frequent passing of urine (polydypsia and polyuria). A random blood glucose test should be routinely performed, if high repeated, then a glucose tolerance test arranged.
- Anxiety – due to the sympathetic neural and hormonal effects patients may develop a dry mouth in conjunction with the other features associated with anxiety. The HAD (hospital anxiety and depression) scale may give an indication of a chronic anxiety state.
- Some patients who complain of a dry mouth have little to show clinically and all investigations are within normal limits. In such cases a delusional state, possibly secondary to a depressive illness, may have developed. Signs and symptoms of this should be sought, such as persistent low mood (more than two weeks), loss of normal interest in things (anhedonia) or poor sleep patterns with typical early-morning waking. The HAD scale may give an insight and appropriate psychological help should be sought.

Table 8-1 **Types of drugs that may produce xerostomia**

- Antidepressants
- Antihistamines
- Anticholinergic drugs
- Potent diuretics
- Hypotensive agents
- Muscle relaxants
- Narcotics
- Hypnotics
- Major tranquillisers
- Sympathomimetics

Increased Salivation (Sialorrhoea)

Increased salivation is common in infants, especially during teething, but is an uncommon complaint during later stages of life. In most cases the condition is transient, usually as a result of stimulation – such as having a painful mouth (for example, mouth ulcers) – or on the initial use of an oral appliance such as in orthodontics or new dentures.

Certain drugs also cause excess salivary production, including anti-cholinesterases, clozapine, cocaine, iodides, bromides, ethyl chloride, dimercaprol, ketamine and digitalis.

In many instances the complaint of excess salivation is not due to a genuine increase but is a result of poor neuromuscular coordination allowing saliva to spill from the mouth or an inability to swallow adequately. This may happen in cerebral palsy, Parkinson's disease, facial palsy and in patients with severe learning disabilities.

Some patients complain of excess salivation for which no local or systemic cause can be identified. This may represent a delusional state that, in turn, may be a manifestation of underlying depressive illness.

Diagnosis
The diagnosis of excess salivation is in essence clinical, although sialometry may be helpful and can be reassuring for the patient whose flow is within normal limits.

Management
Treatment should be directed at the underlying cause, although for many of the neurological problems outlined above this may not be possible. In such instances it may be of value to prescribe medication that has a drying effect. However, other side-effects may make this approach impractical.

For a small number of patients surgical procedures, such as re-routing the submandibular ducts to open more posteriorly or tying off the parotid ducts, can produce symptomatic relief. In patients with a suspected underlying psychological cause appropriate management should be sought. In the case of patients suffering from a delusional state, however, this can be extremely difficult and will almost certainly require specialist psychiatric intervention.

Salivary Gland Infections

Bacteria and viruses can infect the salivary glands.

Mumps

Mumps is an acute febrile illness caused by a paramyxovirus, which is spread by droplet infection. It affects mainly children and young adults. The condition presents with malaise, fever and trismus, followed by a tender swelling of either one or both parotid glands and less frequently the submandibular glands. Mumps usually resolves within a few days and can occasionally be accompanied by non- salivary gland features such as oophoritis, pancreatitis or orchitis. This latter feature is more common in males who develop mumps after puberty and, if bilateral, can result in sterility. Encephalomyelitis is an extremely rare further complication.

Diagnosis
Most cases of mumps can be diagnosed on clinical grounds alone, but the condition can be confirmed by either finding specific antibodies or the virus may be cultured from saliva.

Management
Management tends to be symptomatic with the use of paracetamol, bed rest and ensuring adequate fluid intake. The condition has become less common since the introduction of the measles, mumps and rubella vaccine (MMR).

Recurrent Parotitis of Childhood

This uncommon condition presents with repeated unilateral or bilateral tender swelling of the parotid glands. The cause is unknown and usually the episodes diminish over a period of time.

Diagnosis
This is usually on clinical grounds, although the first episode may be misdiagnosed as mumps. A sialogram may demonstrate the presence of sialectasis.

Management
No specific treatment is available for this condition, with each episode lasting two to three weeks. Symptomatic treatment only may be required.

HIV Salivary Gland Disease

Salivary gland enlargement, most frequently the parotids, can occur as a component of infection with human immunodeficiency virus (HIV). The condition may be accompanied by a dry mouth and is more common when the infection occurs during childhood.

Diagnosis
This condition is unlikely to be the presenting feature of HIV, consequently its diagnosis is most likely clinical. A sialogram may reveal the presence of a sialectasia. Cystic change within the glands may be demonstrable by ultrasound.

Management
Management is largely symptomatic, with the use of artificial saliva if the condition is accompanied by a dry mouth. Lymphoma, not an infrequent complication of HIV disease, may occur in the lymph glands associated with the parotids. This condition needs to be considered if there is a rapid enlargement in the parotid and the relevant investigations (MRI, CT, ultrasound and a needle or core biopsy of the affected tissue arranged). Appropriate management consists of either radiotherapy or chemotherapy.

Suppurative Sialadenitis (Fig 8-4)
This condition can present either sporadically or in association with an existing salivary gland problem such as obstruction (see below) or as a complication of Sjögren's syndrome. The condition presents as an acutely inflamed gland, most frequently the parotid, with pus being expressible from the main duct. The overlying skin may be inflamed and the patient may have an accompanying mild fever.

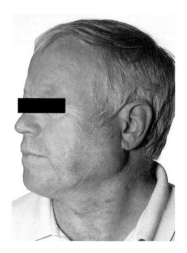

Fig 8-4 Enlargement of left parotid due to acute parotitis. Note how swelling extends under the ear elevating the lobe.

103

Diagnosis
This is usually made on clinical grounds. The presence of an underlying cause, such as the presence of a salivary stone or stricture, should be investigated. The former can be detected on presentation with a plain film or both, when in a non-infective phase, by sialography. Ultrasound may demonstrate the presence of a calculus and associated dilated ducts. Suppurative parotitis can occasionally be more chronic and recurrent, with each episode giving rise to further damage to the gland. This can frequently be demonstrated by sialography, with the presence of ductal dilatation with intermittent narrowing giving rise to a 'string of sausage' appearance where there is associated obstruction (sialodochitis), or sialectasia when there is no associated obstruction.

Management
In the acute phase this is usually by using an antibiotic such as flucloxacillin. If an underlying cause can be found this should be treated accordingly. When the condition recurs on a frequent basis surgical options, such as a partial parotidectomy, may be required.

Salivary Gland Swellings

Mucocele
These occur as a result of a damage to the duct of a minor salivary gland and are most commonly found in the lower lip and floor of mouth. The problem may occur quite suddenly with the development of a dome-shaped, bluish and translucent swelling, which is often asymptomatic. Depending on how deep within the submucosa the condition occurs the problem may remain relatively static or spontaneously burst, releasing mucoid material. The condition can occur at any age.

Mucoceles can be classified on their histological appearance as:
• retention cysts
• extravasation cysts.

Mucous retention cysts have the ductal lining remaining intact around the periphery of the swelling. In mucous extravasation cysts the ductal lining has become ruptured and the resultant wall is formed by granulation tissue. A mucocele in the floor of the mouth associated with the sublingual glands is known as a ranula (Fig 8-5). On rare occasions a ranula can extend around and under the mylohyoid muscle and present as a submandibular swelling known as a plunging ranula.

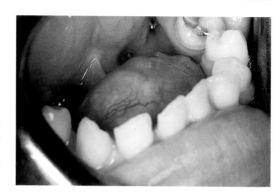

Fig 8-5 Ranula. This translucent sublingual swelling is a result of a mucous retention cyst of the sublingual salivary glands.

Diagnosis

This is usually on clinical grounds, although care should be taken to exclude the possibility of a salivary neoplasm. The general rule is 'swellings in the lower lip are most likely mucoceles whereas those in the upper lip are neoplasms'. An ultrasound examination may help differentiate in cases of doubt, but if there is significant solid component to the swelling a neoplasm should be considered.

Management

Superficial mucoceles may resolve spontaneously, but deeper ones usually require either surgical removal or treatment with cryotherapy.

Sialosis

Sialosis is an asymptomatic enlargement of the salivary glands. It can occur unilaterally or bilaterally and most frequently affects the parotids. The exact cause of this condition is unknown but possibly involves the autonomic innervation of the glands. There may be associated metabolic factors as a result of conditions such as alcoholism, diabetes mellitus or pregnancy or nutritional disorders such as anorexia nervosa or bulimia.

Diagnosis

This is often by exclusion of other causes, although it is asymptomatic and a normal salivary flow rate may be suggestive. Sialography, CT, MRI and ultrasound investigations may be undertaken and will show the presence of a bulky gland with an otherwise normal ductal architecture. A biopsy is usually not required, but underlying causes as indicated above should be investigated.

The condition can occasionally be confused with masseteric hypertrophy, but the latter can usually be determined by the feeling of muscle bulk on clenching or on ultrasound examination. In addition, a diffuse parotid swelling usually causes an elevation of the lobe of the ear.

Management
No specific treatment for this condition is available but it may resolve with management of any underlying systemic factors. Occasionally treatment is sought on cosmetic grounds when a surgical debulking of the gland may be considered.

Sialolithiasis
This condition is the result of a formation of stones (calculi) within the salivary duct. Calculi can be either single or multiple and most frequently occur in the major glands. Those that form in the submandibular ducts are usually well calcified, with concentric layers of calcification. Most that occur in the parotid glands are less well calcified and have a more mucinous texture (mucous plug). The condition characteristically presents with a painful swelling of the affected gland at mealtimes, followed by a slow resolution. In some instances there appears to be little in the way of symptoms, with the resultant stones often reaching considerable size. These are found either by clinical examination or as a chance radiographical finding. The condition tends to affect adults, although occasionally it can occur in childhood. The reason for the calculus formation is unclear but may reflect changes in the composition of the saliva, stasis of salivary flow or the presence of an organic nidus that allows a seeding of calcium salts.

Diagnosis
The presenting complaint is usually diagnostic, although similar features can occur as a result of a ductal stricture or trauma to the orifice. One particular condition affecting the parotid glands occurs as the duct passes through the buccinator muscle where it may be compressed (buccinator window syndrome). Plain film radiographs usually demonstrate the presence of calculi, although those in the parotid may be radiolucent, given that they are often poorly calcified. Ultrasound examination may reveal the presence of the calculus and of the dilatation of the ductal structures proximal to it. Sialography again will demonstrate the presence of the obstruction and, if the contrast can be passed beyond the obstruction, the presence of ductal dilatation and inflammatory change (sialodochitis). Sialography should not be attempted when the calculus can be identified either at the orifice, where it may present as a yellowish swelling, or if the

calculus, as seen by plain film radiography, lies within the floor of mouth. In such situations sialography may push the stone further back along the duct, making retrieval more complex.

Management
This is usually surgical, although for calculi further back in the duct or within the gland it may mean removal of the gland. Asymptomatic calculi within the glands, detected as a chance finding, may be left. Newer techniques, such as lithotripsy and basket retrieval, have been used with some limited success.

Salivary Neoplasms

Both benign and malignant neoplasms can occur in the salivary glands but are relatively rare. They most frequently occur in older adults.

There is a relatively wide variety of salivary neoplasms, and the most frequently used classification is that of the World Health Organization. For further details of this the reader is advised to consult textbooks on oral pathology (see further reading list). The most common benign neoplasm is the pleomorphic salivary adenoma (PSA). The malignant neoplasms include the mucoepidermoid carcinoma and the adenoid cystic carcinoma. The presence of numerous lymph glands associated with the parotid glands means that they are frequently sites for the development of lymphoma.

Tumours of the major salivary glands usually present as a unilateral swelling. In the case of a malignant neoplasm the swelling may progress rapidly. In the parotid such a neoplasm may also involve branches of the facial nerve with associated palsy. With the exception of adenoid cystic carcinoma, lesions are usually relatively asymptomatic. In the case of the benign pleomorphic salivary adenoma the patient may give a history of the swelling being present for many years with only gradual enlargement.

The 'rule of nines' is a rule of thumb that states that nine out of 10 tumours affect the parotid, nine out of 10 are benign and nine out of 10 are pleomorphic salivary adenomas.

Neoplasms affecting minor glands are much less common than those affecting the major glands, with a higher proportion likely to be malignant. Common sites for development are in the upper lip and at the junction of the hard and soft palate.

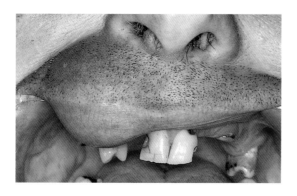

Fig 8-6 Demarcated swelling in upper lip. Such swellings in the upper lip are more likely to be due to neoplasia, and in this case a pleomorphic salivary adenoma.

Pleomorphic Salivary Adenoma (PSA)

This is the most common salivary gland neoplasm (Fig 8-6). It presents as a slow-growing, lobulated, rubbery mass, with the overlying skin or mucosa appearing normal. As it is asymptomatic it can reach a considerable size before presentation. A rapid change in size may indicate the possibility of malignant transformation.

Diagnosis

Initial diagnosis is often on clinical grounds, with imaging modalities such as CT, MRI or ultrasound revealing the presence of an apparently circumscribed lobulated mass with an internal structure that can vary from cyst-like through to dense solid tissue. A pre-operative needle biopsy may help confirm the nature of the condition.

Management

Surgical removal is required with a reasonable margin of surrounding tissue as the lesion is often poorly encapsulated, with the result that, if enucleated, a multifocal recurrence may occur.

Mucoepidermoid Carcinoma

These are usually slow-growing neoplasms and generally of low-grade malignancy. There is a spectrum of disease activity, however, with this neoplasm behaving at times in an almost benign fashion - the other extreme being highly malignant. Its clinical behaviour is difficult to predict histologically.

Diagnosis

As with the pleomorphic salivary adenoma, the mucoepidermoid carcinoma will frequently appear as a defined mass on imaging but is often less circumscribed. A needle biopsy can confirm its histological nature.

Management
Treatment is by surgical excision, with radiotherapy as a possible adjunct.

Adenoid Cystic Carcinoma
This salivary neoplasm can be quite slow-growing but, unlike others, frequently presents with pain, as it has a tendency to perineural spread.

Diagnosis
This is similar as for other salivary neoplasms but on imaging is poorly circumscribed. The clinical picture of pain raises the index of suspicion.

Management
Adenoid cystic carcinoma requires wide surgical resection in view of the perineural spread, which can be at a considerable distance from the main bulk of the neoplasm. The lesion is radio-insensitive and so recurrence is relatively common.

Miscellaneous Salivary Disorders

Necrotising Sialometaplasia (Fig 8-7)
This is a rare benign, self-limiting inflammatory salivary gland disorder. It most frequently occurs in adult males, especially in those who are smokers. The condition occurs as a rapidly developing painless swelling, most frequently around the junction of the hard and soft palate. The swelling rapidly breaks down to form a solitary, often quite deep ulcer with a necrotic base. The condition is self-limiting, usually resolving after several weeks. It appears to be a result of infarction of a minor salivary gland.

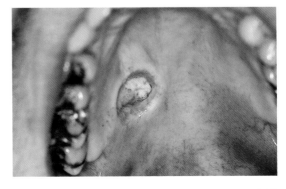

Fig 8-7 Necrotising sialo-metaplasia of the palate, usually seen in smokers, and may be a result of infarction of a minor salivary gland.

Diagnosis
Diagnosis is usually based on clinical features, although a biopsy may help confirm its nature. Occasionally the biopsy may reveal the presence of a pseudoepitheliomatous hyperplasia and lead to a misdiagnosis of a squamous cell carcinoma. Usually clinical features allow differentiation.

Management
As this condition is self-limiting no specific treatment is required, although prevention of secondary infection, using a topical antiseptic such as chlorhexidine, may be of value.

Sarcoidosis
This is a multisystem chronic granulomatous disorder of unknown aetiology. It most commonly affects young adults, and the most frequent presentation is with enlarged hilar lymph nodes in the chest. The parotids may be involved in this condition with swelling (parotitis). For details of other oral manifestations, investigation and management see Chapter 2.

Conclusions

- Salivary gland problems are relatively common.
- The complaint of a dry mouth warrants investigation but may not necessarily be due to an abnormality of the salivary glands.
- Salivary gland disease is a consideration in the differential diagnosis of facial swelling.
- A number of benign and malignant neoplasms can affect the salivary glands, but most are rare.

Further Reading

Pedlar J, Frame JW Oral and Maxillofacial Surgery. London: Churchill Livingstone, 2001 (pp.195-210).

Scully C, Flint SR, Porter SR. Oral Diseases. London: Martin Dunitz, 1996.

Soames JV, Southam JC. Oral Pathology 4th ed. Oxford: Oxford Medical Publications, 2005.

Chapter 9
Facial Pain

Aim

This chapter aims to make the clinical pattern of different pain problems more recognisable and highlights the importance of using quality of life as a measure of success.

Outcome

After reading this chapter you should be able to see the patient behind the pain, to form an appropriate differential diagnosis and treatment plan to obtain the best improvement in quality of life.

Chronic Facial Pain

This section is concerned with chronic facial pain still present once dental and non-dental pathological conditions have been excluded. Pain appreciation can have many triggers, the simplest of which is central or peripheral nerve damage (neuropathic pain). Similarly, when nerve function is changed by an alteration in neurotransmitter balance, synaptic signal transmission is also altered and thus the appreciation of information by the nervous system changes. Both somatic and autonomic pathways pass information to the brain for consideration. Thus damage or alteration to either or both of these can lead to pain appreciation by the individual. In addition, dysfunction of nerves that have a motor or vasomotor 'component' can produce changes in the tissues detected by the patient. This is most commonly seen in the autonomic system, where vasomotor changes accompany pain in many individuals, leading them to report swelling, erythema or sweating in the region affected by the pain.

Understanding Pain

The idea that pain is a simple stimulus and response system as proposed by Descartes is now rarely voiced. In fact, pain as 'a sensation' is in question. There are undoubtedly pathways in the nervous system responsible for the transmission of damage signals from the tissues. It is the appreciation and interpretation of this information within the brain that results in the perception of pain. If pain is considered a 'state of mind' rather than a pure sensation it is easier to understand how many of the chronic pain conditions can arise when little or no tissue damage is evident. Alteration of the chemical balance of the brain, be it by damage signals from the tissues, emotional changes or drug therapy can all change perception of pain and the pattern or type of signals into the brain that can be interpreted as pain. Pain is now considered multidimensional. It is defined by the International Association for the Study of Pain as 'an unpleasant sensory and emotional experience, associated with actual or potential tissue damage, or described in terms of such damage'. This reflects both the patient's experience that pain is often triggered by tissue damage and the clinician's, that mood and pain perception are intimately linked.

Allodynia

Tissue damage releases chemical mediators that activate both A delta and C fibres. These mediators also lower the threshold sensitivity of the pain nerves, making further firing possible with a lower level of stimulation. Chronic nerve stimulation can therefore lead to such a lowering of the firing thresholds that innocuous triggers, including normal sensation, can be enough to cause the pain nerves to fire. Injury to sensory nerves also triggers nerve 'sprouting'. This results in new connections forming in the dorsal horn of the spinal cord from somatic sensory nerves to pain fibres after sensory nerve injury. Stimulation of the sensory nerve then causes the pain pathways in the spinal cord to activate inappropriately. The effect of both changes is to promote chronic pain in previously damaged tissue without any ongoing damage. This is known as allodynia.

Pain Appreciation

Even with activation of the A delta and C fibres, pain transmission to the brain is not guaranteed. The 'Gate Theory' proposed by Melzak and Wall suggested that other nerve activity within the spinal column could modulate the passage of the pain signals to the brain. This can either inhibit transmission, as with the battlefield casualty unaware of an injury, or facilitate pain as seen in an anxious patient undergoing operative dental care. The control of pain transmission and appreciation by the higher centres is very important in clinical practice, with the brain having the ability to block or facilitate pain appreciation. The anxious patient can even feel true pulpal pain by activation of pain memories by Pavlovian association before the tooth has been touched.

Phantom limb pain provides a clear example that nerve signals from the body are not necessary for pain to be 'felt', demonstrating that pain as well as all other sensations are literally 'in the mind' rather than localised to a body part. When looking at methods for controlling chronic pain it is important to consider both central and peripherally acting drugs, psychological and physical treatments. All have a role to play. In many cases of chronic pain there may be more than one 'pain' problem acting together, and this may require a combination approach to treatment – partly mood and psychological therapy and in part drug or physical treatments.

Neurogenic and Vascular Facial Pain

This section includes a variety of clinical presentations where it appears that normal nerve function is disrupted, leading to the perception of pain. These conditions are listed in Table 9-1.

Pain without Vasomotor Changes

Trigeminal Neuralgia
Trigeminal neuralgia (TN) is a well-recognised condition affecting predominantly older patients. It is a common condition presenting over the winter months. The exact prevalence is not known, but is thought to be in the order of six per million population, with a slight female predisposition.

Table 9-1 **Neurogenic Facial Pain**

- Pain without vasomotor changes
  - Trigeminal neuralgia
  - Stroke pain
  - Neuropathic pain
  - Atypical odontalgia

- Pain with vasomotor changes
  - Migrainous neuralgia
  - Complex regional pain syndrome

It is an extremely debilitating condition for the affected individuals, with sudden-onset, short-duration, high-intensity, lancinating or 'electric shock-type' pain. This radiates from a focal point or 'trigger zone' in the trigeminal distribution and is severe enough to halt the patient's activities abruptly. The pain usually passes in seconds, but its severity causes the patient to adopt a variety of strategies to try to prevent the pain returning. Most often trigeminal neuralgia involves the mandibular or maxillary divisions and is unilateral. Variations exist, however, with bilateral pain or a persisting burning pain in the trigger area after the initial sudden burst reported by some patients. It is essential to perform a cranial nerve examination for all patients presenting with TN. There should be no neurological deficit detected, but occasionally problems are found. Common findings include trigeminal sensory loss or marked deafness on the pain side. In these circumstances, or when a patient younger than 50 is suspected of having TN, the clinician should be suspicious about the presence of central nervous system (CNS) disease. An MRI examination is then essential and may identify a focal or diffuse brain lesions, such as an acoustic nerve neuroma or multiple sclerosis.

The trigger and mechanism for the pain in TN remains unclear. There is no evidence to support a peripheral nerve dysfunction. An abnormality of nerve signal-processing within the CNS seems more likely, perhaps due to compression of the nerve root at the trigeminal ganglion.

Treatment of TN is initially medical, and most patients respond well to carbamazepine therapy. This medication does have some disadvantages, however, including causing an allergic rash in some. In the elderly population, who most frequently present with TN, the drug side-effects can be very limiting. Sedation, cerebellar and balance disorders together with alterations to liver drug metabolism can all lead to dose limitations or early termination of treatment and consequently the return of the pain. The use of the modified release preparation of carbamazepine can minimise some of these effects. When an alternative medical treatment is required, gabapentin, baclofen, phenytoin, oxcarbazapine and lamotrigine have all been used with success. Occasionally it is necessary to combine one or more drug treatments to get adequate pain relief. Patients with multiple sclerosis can be particularly resistant to conventional therapy but may respond to high-dose systemic corticosteroids. Surgical care has traditionally been reserved for patients for whom medical treatments had failed. However, early surgical intervention is now thought to be an advantage by eliminating the need for medication or, more commonly, reducing the dose required for adequate pain control. Operative morbidity and mortality may also be reduced by treating patients while they are younger and fitter. However, destructive peripheral nerve surgery, such as an alcohol nerve block of the affected trigeminal branch, should now only be performed as a palliative procedure. These procedures ultimately cause allodynia, making the pain problem worse, and should be reserved for patients both unable to tolerate effective medical therapy and unfit for other CNS surgical procedures. Retrogasserian glycerol injection and radiofrequency thermocoagulation of the trigeminal ganglion are destructive neurosurgical procedures that would be expected to leave the patient with hemifacial anaesthesia on the operated side. Surprisingly, light touch is often preserved, although patients do report altered sensation and they tolerate the procedure remarkably well. Vascular decompression procedures around the trigeminal ganglion have met with a high degree of success but with a higher operative risk. At present they seem the best surgical option for the younger patient.

Stroke Pain

A cerebrovascular accident or stroke is a brain injury that leads to a permanent loss of motor, sensory or cognitive function. Although the brain itself has no pain awareness, damage to parts of the brain involved in pain appreciation can result in altered perception of pain. This can lead the individual to experience pain without a nociceptive input, and in some patients facial or dental pain can result. The time between the onset of the pain and the stroke is the key to the diagnosis. Treatment strategies outlined below for neuropathic pain are the most helpful in managing this difficult condition, but often a full range of pain strategies needs to be employed.

Neuropathic Pain

The term 'neuropathic' pain implies damage to nerves that leads to altered transmission of normal signals from the tissues to the CNS. These altered signals are then interpreted as pain. Some nerve injury conditions are well known to predispose a patient to chronic pain. These include damage resulting from *Herpes zoster* reactivation (shingles), alcohol nerve block (anaesthesia dolorosa) or even damage to the inferior alveolar nerve during third-molar surgery. In many cases, though, this damage is not significant and pain may follow an apparently successful minor surgical procedure, such as an apicectomy or even an uneventful extraction. Here, the prolonged postoperative discomfort may be misdiagnosed as persisting infection, leading to repeated surgery, which only exacerbates the nerve damage and increases the pain.

Rarely is the pain from neuropathic damage severe. It may cause significant disability, however, due to its unremitting nature and can become a destructive force in the patient's life. There is increasing evidence that some patients are prone to developing such damage due to inherited variations to their nerve ion channels. This understanding may lead to more specific and targeted treatments in the future.

Often neuropathic pain is described as a burning feeling in the tissues and it is well localised by the patient. Typically the discomfort is present on waking, continues all of the day but does not prevent sleep at night. There is some day-to-day variation in the intensity of symptoms but no specific relationship to routine daily activities or oral function. At present the best initial treatment is medical, with gabapentin and valproate proving the most useful agents. These can be combined with a tricyclic drug such as amitriptyline. Physical treatment has a role to play in neuropathic pain, however, particularly low-frequency TENS and acupuncture. In most patients treatment continues for many years, but it is worth periodically reassessing the management strategy.

Atypical Odontalgia

This condition is most likely due to neuropathic damage involving the mechanisms associated with pulpal sensory information leading into the CNS. It produces intense pain indistinguishable from an acute pulpitis. This frequently leads to endodontics and ultimately extraction of teeth in one particular region of the mouth. There is no method of easily separating patients with atypical odontalgia from those with other causes of pulpitis, other than elimination of possible dental disease. Obviously, this can prove difficult in the heavily restored tooth. When extraction is carried out, the pain is usually relieved for a few weeks, but eventually it returns again in an adjacent tooth or in the extraction site. Medical treatments used for neuropathic pain are often helpful in reducing the symptoms in atypical odontalgia. As the pain is truly 'toothache', most patients with this condition eventually seek extraction of the painful tooth despite their awareness that this rarely solves the problem. It is sensible for this to be accepted by the clinician so that a professional relationship with the patient can be maintained. Developing an agreed strategy for management of acute pain episodes, including the use of opioid analgesics and ultimately planned extractions, will usually slow the progress towards edentulousness.

Pain with Vasomotor Changes

In some patients with chronic pain there is an alteration to the blood flow to a painful area that is not related to its metabolic need. This seems to be as a result of sympathetic nerve dysfunction, and normal control over the arterial blood supply is lost. The stellate ganglion supplies the entire head and neck with sympathetic nerves. As a consequence the area that can be affected by the vasomotor changes is both large and diffuse. Even if the site of pain and the vasomotor effects differ in the head or face, the onset of pain and vasomotor changes at the same time suggests that they are connected. The most common vasomotor changes reported by patients include a feeling of pressure or tissue-swelling, erythema of the skin, nasal congestion (nasal mucosal swelling), lacrimation and diffuse and inappropriate head and neck sweating.

Migrainous Neuralgia

Migrainous neuralgia or 'cluster headache' is a relatively uncommon but disabling condition of unknown aetiology. It is characterised by an intense unilateral headache that may extend onto or exclusively involve the face. It usually has a sudden onset and settles spontaneously after several hours. Many patients report that the attacks occur at the same time each day, but without any obvious trigger. The attacks usually last for about six weeks before settling spontaneously. The patient may then be painfree for many months until, without warning, the pain returns and another 'cluster' begins (episodic cluster headache). Some patients have identical symptoms but do not get any remission, having this debilitating problem on most days over many years (chronic cluster headache). Accompanying the pain are characteristic vasomotor changes, with lacrimation and nasal congestion most often being reported by patients. A feeling of swelling and erythema of the painful area are also common.

There are no investigations that are helpful, and the diagnosis is usually made from the pattern of pain given in the history. Treatment for patients with episodic and chronic cluster variants differs, as in the latter there is the opportunity for prophylactic medication. In episodic cluster headache it is usual to treat each attack at the onset and wait for the cluster to pass. Here the most useful drugs are the 5-HT agonists, such as sumatriptan and zolmatriptan. Patient-administered injections or sublingual drug absorption have good response rates, and these are preferred at present over oral preparations. In chronic cluster headache preventative therapy is desirable due to the unremitting nature of the attacks, and gabapentin, verapamil and lithium have all been found useful in some patients. Other treatments have been suggested, including high–dose systemic steroid regimens, high-flow oxygen and intranasal lignocaine spray. These are undoubtedly helpful in some patients, but often the successful treatment for an individual patient is found by trial and error.

Complex Regional Pain Syndrome

Complex regional pain syndrome (CRPS) is a recent term introduced to describe patients with specific patterns of pain, usually affecting one body region, such as a limb, where the pain is accompanied by a variety of other symptoms. It is thought to be related to low-level nerve damage. Previously the term reflex sympathetic dystrophy (RSD) was used for this condition. In many ways it can be thought of as a neuropathic pain affecting the sympathetic nerves in a body region. As these nerves are both afferent and efferent, the symptoms described reflect this with pain (afferent) and vasomotor changes (efferent) in the involved region. This produces the complex symptomatology these patients describe and, as a consequence, many patients with CRPS were previously labeled as 'atypical facial pain', as the symptoms did not seem to make sense. As with neuropathic pain, a genetic predisposition to develop pain seems to be present in patients with CRPS. Innocuous trauma can lead to quite marked symptoms and disability. Patients with CRPS often have very delocalised unilateral or bilateral pain over the face, head and neck, not respecting the 'normal' anatomical boundaries of the somatic nerve divisions. The pain is described as burning or gripping and follows a similar pattern to neuropathic pain, with day-to-day variation in the pain intensity without specific precipitating or relieving factors. Drug therapy has had limited success, with gabapentin, sodium valproate and lamotrigine being the most useful agents. These drugs all act on the GABA receptor family, and it may be that newer drugs acting on these receptors will be useful in the future. Acupuncture can also be useful in these patients but requires long-term treatment. New therapies are being tried as the pathophysiology of the injured nerve is better understood, and NMDA-blocking drugs, such as amantidine and the antiarrhythmics mexilitine and tocainamide or their derivatives, may prove useful in the future.

Headache

Most patients seen in a hospital setting with chronic headache attend neurology clinics. An increasing awareness of the possible role for the oral and dental structures in some forms of headache, however, has led to a rise in the numbers of referrals to dental specialties. A useful classification for headaches is given in Table 9-2, and a fuller overview listed in the further reading at the end of this chapter.

All patients presenting with headache must have a full neurological assessment, as intracranial lesions and some degenerative changes can present as a headache. If there is any doubt that the patient is not fully neurologically

Table 9-2 **Headache Classification** (modified from Headache and Facial Pain, Richard Peatfield, in Medicine Vol 32, issue 9, 2004)

Recurrent headaches	Migraine Cluster headache Episodic tension headache
Triggered headache	Coughing, straining, exertion Coitus Food and drink
Dull headache increasing in severity	Usually benign Overuse of medication (codeine) Contraceptive pill, hormone replacement therapy Neck disease Temporal arteritis Benign intracranial hypertension Cerebral tumour
Dull headache unchanged over months	Chronic tension headache Temperomandibular disorder Depressive headache

intact, an MRI scan is essential to exclude intracranial pathology and an appropriate referral made to a neurologist. Headaches presenting to the dental specialties include:

- classical migraine
- common migraine
- tension-type headache
- temporal arteritis
- temporomandibular disorders

Classical Migraine

Migraine sufferers usually have an intense unilateral headache that is associated with nausea, photophobia and hyperacusis, although bilateral symptoms are not unusual. Classical migraine presents with an 'aura' or warning of the onset of the pain and associated symptoms. During the aura the patient may see flashing lights or lines (fortification lines), but it can produce other sensory perceptions, including a particular taste or smell. During the aura many patients obtain relief from simple preparations such as paracetamol, caffeine and anti-emetic-based drugs. Others will deteriorate and can be significantly disabled by their symptoms for several days. For these patients, or those with at least two major episodes monthly, preventative treatments can be helpful. Discovering the most effective regimen from the very long list of possibilities is often a matter of trial and error, but some patients are never able to find an acceptable treatment. EEG studies suggest that the changes leading to migraine pain may start some days before the actual pain begins. Preventative treatments must therefore be continuous to be effective. If a patient does not have frequent attacks, therapy at the beginning of each pain period is more appropriate. Episodic treatment has been revolutionised by the 'triptan' drugs, such as zolmatriptan, which can be given sublingually at the onset of an attack and repeated, if necessary, after two hours. The sublingual route allows for rapid action and is unaffected by the nausea or vomiting associated with migraine attacks.

Common Migraine
When a patient presents with all the symptoms of classical migraine but without the associated aura or prodromal features, this is termed 'common' migraine and is managed in the same manner as classical migraine.

Tension Type Headache
This is a common condition often described by the patient as a feeling of pressure or a tight band around the head. The symptoms can be very variable, however, with unilateral, bilateral, anterior or posterior cranial symptoms. Tension-type headache is similar to temperomandibular dysfunction (TMD) in its demographics and symptom description. There is often considerable overlap between these conditions where patients presenting with TMD will also report cranial, neck and shoulder pain. Both of these conditions show a significant relationship to stress. Management of tension-type headache can be through cognitive behavioral therapy and simple analgesics. In some cases tricyclic-based drugs are helpful, offering anxiolysis, muscle relaxation and a reduction in pain perception.

Temporal Arteritis

This condition must not be overlooked in any consideration of facial pain. Temporal arteritis (sometimes called cranial arteritis) is a vasculitic disorder of unknown cause. It is discussed in Chaper 2.

Temporomandibular Disorders

Patients with pain in the region of the temporomandibular joints (TMJ) are common and often considered as a single group, leading to inappropriate management of most. The most basic differentiation for patients reporting pain around the TMJ is between those with joint pathology, such as a meniscal tear, and those without joint pathology. A crude method of separating these groups is from a history of joint-locking, suggesting significant internal TMJ derangement. Patients with obvious meniscal damage are best assessed by a surgeon with an interest in the temporomandibular joint. They are investigated with MRI imaging of the TMJ and ultimately arthroscopy to determine the need for surgical repair. Symptoms such as clicking or crepitus from the joint are common both with and without significant meniscal damage and are therefore poor discriminators for surgical rather than medical referral.

The remaining patients with pain in the TMJ region are better termed temporomandibular dysfunction (TMD), which does not imply any joint pathology, while at the same time acknowledging the localisation of the pain to the lateral aspect of the face, head and neck. TMD can present at any age, mimicking toothache in children, being found during periods of examinations or relationship stress in the young adult, in association with difficult social or family circumstances in the middle-aged and with bereavement or anticipation of an uncertain future in the elderly. Many of these groups require tailored interventions, but those affected in each age group share certain characteristics, particularly a tendency towards an anxiety neurosis. It is important to emphasise that success in treatment with TMD patients depends largely upon the patient. Patients must accept responsibility for their own care, as most treatments are suggested by the physician but implemented by the patient. Consequently, the patient who is unwilling to fully cooperate with a treatment plan rarely has a successful outcome. Simple measures can be used successfully in patients with TMD problems. Cognitive techniques, such as explaining the condition and its natural history of relapses and exacerbations, together with reassurance about the absence of serious disease, may be all that is required initially. Combining this with a bite splint is successful at relieving symptoms in the majority of patients with TMD pain. Despite many claims to the contrary there is no 'best design'. Most forms of bite-opening, repositioning, upper or lower appliances are successful in most patients. There are always anecdotal stories of particular patients or practitioners who have success with one variant or another, but for the majority of TMD patients a simple, cheap, easy-to-fit and, importantly, an easy-to-wear appliance is adequate. There is little role for physical therapies such as physiotherapy or acupuncture in the initial management of chronic TMD. Such physical treatments do give a good short-term symptom improvement in most patients, but this is not sustained at the end of treatment, as the underlying problems often remain. However, they can be very useful in converting acute TMD pain into a chronic form, which allows for conventional treatment.

In patients where splint therapy has not produced good resolution within two months, longer splint wear by itself will be of little additional benefit. In many studies it has been shown that the combination of a splint with a tricyclic-based drug such as amitriptyline is more beneficial than use of a splint alone. These drugs are anxiolytic and relaxant and when taken at night seem to positively influence sleep patterns and reduce pain perception in the brain. If continued for some months after symptoms have resolved the pain relapse rate is reduced. Where the TMD symptoms are part of a generalised pain disorder the early use of tricyclics and cognitive therapy seem particularly helpful. This includes patients reporting irritable bowel syndrome, chronic non-ulcer dyspepsia, neck and shoulder pain or fibromyalgia.

Acute TMD pain can be very unpleasant and distressing for the patient. Usually there is a clear history of relapsing chronic TMD, but the presenting pain may be described more as a 'toothache' or an 'abscess' by the patient. Always consider the possibility of TMD pain in a patient presenting with acute 'dental' pain and routinely ask about previous TMD symptoms when taking the history. A local anaesthetic injection in the upper third molar region will relieve the discomfort in most acute TMD patients and can be helpful in establishing the diagnosis. The aim of treatment in acute TMD is to convert the symptoms from acute pain to chronic pain so that 'standard' TMD interventions can be used. Therapy should begin with a strict soft diet, muscle relaxants such as diazepam, and a potent NSAID taken regularly for a period of about two weeks. At this stage physiotherapy and acupuncture can be also be effective in reducing the patient's symptoms.

Oral Dysaesthesias

These conditions are changes in perception of the oral environment rather than a disease. Dysaesthesias can be thought of as 'pins and needles' of the oral special sensory apparatus, although this is not true in reality. They are part of a range of somatisation disorders seen in patients and frequently coexist with problems such as irritable bowel syndrome and chronic non-ulcer dyspepsia. This does not imply that all patients with dysaesthesias have a psychiatric diagnosis. There are patients with no psychological problems who clearly have a dysaesthesia, and it seems that the perceptual alteration in the brain is primarily a biochemical change. This can be driven by different factors, including, but not exclusively, the anxiety states often seen in chronic somatisers. Dysaesthesias can affect any sensory modality in the mouth or face, with the patient reporting changes in moisture (dry mouth or hypersalivation), thermal sensation (burning mouth), taste (dysgeusia), smell (halitosis) or normal sensation (hypoaesthesia). It is very important to remember that these symptoms can also indicate disease, and a dysaesthesia can only be diagnosed once all tissue and CNS pathologies have been excluded. Some suspected dysaesthesias can be confirmed by clinical observation, such as the perception of a dry mouth in the presence of copious saliva, but on occasions more invasive tests, such as haematinic estimation, biochemical tests, immunological assays, radiography and MRI may be needed. It may be also be necessary for the patient to consult colleagues from periodontology or ENT to eliminate focal infection as a possible cause for a perceived bad taste or smell. On occasions treatments such as systemic antifungal medication may be used to eliminate the possibility of fungal infection as the cause of a burning dysaesthesia, or a trial of iron supplements may be needed in patients found to have low ferritin levels. Some conditions such as dysaesthesic dryness or burning seem more commonly associated with anxiety disorders than the others. In these patients a pharyngeal tightness or a 'globus sensation' is often reported by the patient. It is very important to take a full medical and social history for patients with dysaesthesias, as many have health or home stressors contributing to their problem. One characteristic feature of dysaesthesic symptoms is their distractability, with other oral activities relieving the patient's awareness of their problem. A good example of this is the loss of awareness of the 'burning mouth' when eating. Although many patients find their symptoms to be only irritating, some become significantly disabled in their oral function and quality of life. The most reliable treatments for those with no haematinic deficiency or fungal infection have been based around anxiolytics, including tricyclic drugs such as amitriptyline. The different dysaesthesias, however, show differing tendencies to resolve, with dryness and burning being the most responsive and taste and smell changes the least. Clinical psychology intervention can give similar results and is particularly helpful where only a partial response is obtained to medical therapy or where significant social problems exist to drive the condition onwards.

Summary

- Chronic facial pain can lead to a poor quality of life in many patients.

- The history must be taken carefully – the diagnosis will be there.
- Neuropathic pain and CRPS can be the result of minimal injury in susceptible patients.
- TMD must always be considered as a cause of acute or chronic facial pain.
- Pain is always 'in the mind' but rarely imagined.

Further Reading

Orofacial Pain
Zakrzewska JM, Harrison SD (eds) Pain Research and Clinical Management Vol 14 – Assessment and Management of Orofacial Pain London: Elsevier, 2002.

Ghali GE, Epker BN. Clinical neurosensory testing: practical applications. J Oral Maxillofac Surg 1989;47:10,1074-1078.

Trigeminal Neuralgia
Zakrzewska JM .Trigeminal Neuralgia (Major Problems in Neurology) London: Saunders, 1995.

Headache Management
The International Classification of Headache Disorders, 2nd Edition. Cephalgia 2004; 24:Suppl 1.

Rozen TD. Antiepileptic drugs in the management of cluster headache and trigeminal neuralgia. Headache 2001;41:Suppl 1:S25-32.

Temporomandibular Disorders
Koh H, Robinson PG. Occlusal adjustment for treating and preventing temporomandibular joint disorders. Cochrane Database Syst Rev 2003;1.

Schwartz M, Freund B. Treatment of temporomandibular disorders with botulinum toxin. Clin J Pain. 2002;18:6,Suppl:S198-203.

Oral Dyasaesthesia
Friedlander AH, Friedlander IK, Gallas M, Velasco E. Late-life depression: its oral health significance. Int Dent J 2003;53:1,41-50.

Scala A, Checchi L, Montevecchi M et al. Update on burning mouth syndrome: overview and patient management. Crit Rev Oral Biol Med 2003;14:4,275-291.

Zakrzewska JM, Glenny AM, Forssell H. Interventions for the treatment of burning mouth syndrome. Cochrane Database Syst Rev 2001;3.

Chapter 10
Neurological Disorders of the Head and Neck

Aim

This chapter reviews the common neurological problems that may present in the head and neck.

Outcome

After reading this chapter you should be able to describe the presenting features of common neurological conditions in the head, neck and mouth.

Introduction

Brain structure and function rarely feature prominently in the dental curriculum, but a knowledge of some basic features is helpful in understanding why patients can present with particular symptoms in particular conditions.

The cerebral cortex is the controlling centre in the brain, which initiates voluntary actions in the body and processes the sensory information flowing in from the peripheral nervous system. Between these two are a variety of brain areas that process and modify the information flowing into and away from the cortex. Dysfunction of specific brain areas gives symptoms with characteristic clinical patterns. One function of the cerebellum, for example, is to control and modify fine movement, therefore lesions in this area produce a tremor on voluntary movements but not at rest. Lesions in the substantia nigra, on the other hand, produce a tremor at rest that is lost on movement, predominantly seen in the limbs but also evident in the mandible.

Most of the cranial nerves leave the brain in the pons and the medulla. Lesions here will have orofacial consequences - for example, a facial weakness following a stroke. Some of the cranial nerves run close together in their intracranial course, and pathology of one may affect another. A neuroma of the acoustic nerve (VIII) can produce symptoms in the trigeminal (V) and the facial (VII) nerves. Thus the patient presenting to the clinician with unilateral facial weakness or numbness should be checked for deafness on the same side, which could suggest such a lesion.

Testing the cranial nerves is an important clinical skill, which can be mastered easily by all medical and dental practitioners. A basic test can be performed in less than a minute by an experienced practitioner (Table 10-1).

Neuromuscular problems of the head and neck of importance to the dental clinician include the following:
• movement disorders
• sensory loss
• motor loss.

Movement Disorders

Movement disorders involving the head and neck can make delivery of dental care difficult. Knowledge of the type of movement disorder and an appreciation that the patient has little or no control over the problem are important. The movement disorders of importance are:
• Cerebral palsy
• Parkinson's disease.

Cerebral Palsy

Cerebral palsy is characterised by a fixed neurological defect that is thought to occur around the time of birth. This condition affects each individual in a different way, with some having only motor control problems and others having cognitive impairment as well. It is important to realise that many patients with cerebral palsy are of normal intelligence. They have a problem with control of movement, often exacerbated by limb spasticity. In others there are writhing (athetotic) motions of the limbs at rest, which often become worse if the patient is sedated or concentrating on remaining still.

Parkinson's Disease

This is a widespread degenerative movement disorder characterised by a difficulty in initiating movement and a marked limb tremor at rest. In many patients this tremor reduces significantly when purposeful movements are made. Patients often have difficulty in initiating movements, moving through doorways and in starting to speak. This leaves what seems like an 'awkward pause' before they reply to questions, but the patient should be given the necessary time to respond. Head and neck involvement can cause purposeless mandibular movements at rest. These usually disappear when the patient holds their mouth open for treatment. Many patients are unaware

Table 10-1 **Quick Chairside Cranial Nerve Examination**

Nerve	Name	Test
I	Olfactory	Not usually tested in the limited examination
II	Optic	Test each eye separately Can count fingers held 1m in front of the patient Visual fields tested by moving object into vision from four distinct points in the periphery with the patient's gaze straight ahead Pupillary reflex contraction to light and dilation to close visual accommodation bilaterally (requires intact III)
III	Occulomotor	Tested with IV and VI Each eye can track a moving object smoothly up, down, left and right. When the eyes are tested together no double vision is reported near to the extremes of gaze or looking straight ahead Eyelid retraction occurs with upward gaze Pupillary responses listed in II also require intact III function.
IV	Trochlear	Tested with III Lesion produces weakness in upward and outward gaze on the affected side only
V	Trigeminal	Sensory to the face Test light touch and pinprick sensation (with cotton wool and a blunted needle) to each of the trigeminal branches on each side of the face Motor to the masticatory muscles Get the patient to clench the teeth onto an object (wood spatula) on first one side, then the other, with the examiner trying to remove the object each time
VI	Abducent	Tested with III. Lesion prevents lateral gaze on the affected side only

VII	Facial	Motor to the facial muscles Get the patient to: - raise their brow - tightly shut the eyes - make a pout with the lips
VIII	Acoustic	Hearing Cover one ear, whisper a word into the open ear and ask the patient to repeat the word. Repeat for the other ear Balance Stand the patient upright with their eyes closed and gently push the patient to one side. Balance should be maintained. If not, be prepared to steady the patient
IX	Glossopharyngeal	Tested with X Touch the back of the soft palate with an instrument. The patient should retch and elevate the soft palate
X	Vagus	Tested with IX
XI	Accessory	Get the patient to elevate their shoulders and then turn their head to each side against resistance provided by the examiner
XII	Hypopglossal	Get the patient to protrude the tongue. There should be no deviation to the side. If there is, the tongue deviates towards the weak side

of their movements at rest. Initially the symptoms can be well controlled with dopaminergic agonists and monoamine oxidase inhibitor drugs, but this control is gradually lost as the disease progresses. These drugs reduce salivary flow, and most patients complain about a dry mouth.

Other degenerative movement disorders, such as those related to drug treatments (tardive diskinesias) or alcohol abuse, do not improve with medical treatment and pose an increasing challenge to the treating dentist.

Sensory Disorders

Facial sensory loss is a very important symptom and should provoke the clinician into a structured investigation to determine the cause. It is essential to determine in the history whether an episode of sensory loss has occurred previously, either in the face or elsewhere in the body and whether the symptoms have been of gradual or sudden onset. A full cranial nerve examination should follow and any area of sensory change mapped out, noting which sensory modalities are changed – light touch, pinprick and thermal are the most easily tested. Firm pressure sensation often remains, although the mechanism for this is not clear. The likely cause of the problem is related to the rapidity of onset of the sensory change as detailed in Table 10-2. The clin-

Table 10-2 **Facial Sensory Loss**

Gradual onset	Intracranial tumour – for example, acoustic neuroma, astrocytoma - unilateral loss for pons and above - bilateral loss possible for brainstem and spinal cord
	Syringobulbia - often bilateral changes anteriorly in the face
	Midface tumour - for example, maxillary sinus giving maxillary sensory loss
	Drug reactions - rarely found in drugs causing peripheral neuropathy
	Diabetes mellitus - peripheral neuropathy associated with microvascular disease
Sudden onset	Local anaesthetic
	Trauma to sensory nerves (including facial bone fractures)
	Infection along the nerve course - V maxillary or mandibular branch involvement in a dentoalveolar abscess
	Intracranial infection - for example, HSV encephalopathy
	Multiple sclerosis - usually multiple divisions unilateral
	Cerebral bleed or infarction (stroke)
	Benign trigeminal neuropathy

ician's knowledge of facial and neuro-anatomy will help to determine where the lesion is likely to be found. It is then important to arrange appropriate investigations. In particular it is essential to eliminate any local focal dental or facial cause or a cerebrovascular infarction before considering less common possibilities such as multiple sclerosis and intracranial tumours. Bilateral facial sensory loss is often taken as suggesting a psychiatric problem, but true bilateral sensory loss can occur as a result of lesions in the spinal nucleus of the trigeminal nerve. Dilatation of the brain stem and spinal CSF canal (syringobulbia) can lead to this presentation. In some patients no cause is identified for their facial sensory loss, and it gradually resolves. These cases are usually labelled 'benign trigeminal neuropathy', and the problem does not seem to be recurrent. It may be the result of trigeminal ganglion inflammation, as focal demyleination of the ganglion is seen on MRI scan in some patients. The cause is not clear, but infection by a herpes group virus has been suggested in view of its association with the trigeminal nerve.

Intracranial Disease

Lesions in the CNS that interrupt normal nerve function can present as facial sensory loss. Space-occupying lesions (usually tumours) produce their symptoms gradually and present with a worsening clinical picture over time. Of special interest here is the acoustic neuroma, sometimes referred to as the cerebello-pontine angle tumour in view of its location. This benign tumour produces a swelling on the acoustic (VIII) nerve where it is in close proximity to the trigeminal (V) and facial nerves (VII). The patient may complain of progressive unilateral loss of facial sensation and often weakness of the muscles of mastication on the same side. This condition is identified during a cranial nerve examination, as the patient's hearing will have been lost on the same side due to the direct effects of the tumour on the acoustic nerve. Infarction of brain tissue, often referred to as a cerebrovascular accident (CVA) or stroke, can produce sensory as well as motor changes and is the most common cause for sensory loss in the body. Inflammatory changes in the brain are found in lupus and other connective tissue diseases and other immunologically mediated conditions, such as coeliac disease, and therefore can also be associated with facial sensory loss.

Multiple Sclerosis

This is a degenerative disorder of the myelin covering of the nerves within the central nervous system. Its cause remains unknown, but it seems that there are both genetic and environmental factors involved. Women are more likely to contract the condition than men. It progresses over many years with gradual functional impairment of sensory, motor, autonomic and cognitive function. The rate of progression varies between individuals and with time. Often there are periods of disease activity with deterioration, interspersed with remissions for months or years. The degree of final disability is very variable. Some patients succumb to the effects of the neuronal degeneration and others experience only minor impairments in their everyday life. An early presenting feature is that of sudden sensory loss in part of the body. This can involve cutaneous sensation, such as in the face, or special sensation, such as vision. Within a few weeks function has returned to normal, with no apparent residual deficit to the patient. Even after apparent recovery, however, the nerve damage remains and can be measured by studying nerve response times, such as visual evoked potentials or conduction velocity testing. A patient presenting with sudden onset facial or oral sensory loss should be questioned about similar episodes in the face, elsewhere in the body or visual changes that may have recovered after a few weeks. The typical patient presenting with MS is a woman aged 20 to 35 with sudden hemifacial sensory loss with neither a history of trauma nor any local cause found. MS is strongly suspected if plaques of demyelination are seen in the brain on a MRI scan and, following this, the patient should be referred to a neurologist to have the diagnosis confirmed. There is no treatment for the sensory loss and in most patients it will resolve within a few weeks. Patients with MS are prone to trigeminal neuralgia and MS must be considered for a younger patient presenting with typical trigeminal neuralgia pain.

Facial Motor Loss

This problem is most often confined to the facial nerve (VII), although isolated palsies of other facial and ocular movements are occasionally seen. Masticatory muscle weakness together with facial sensory loss can be found when the trigeminal nerve has been damaged along its intracranial or extracranial course. Multiple motor palsies are sometimes found in patients with intracranial damage, HIV, intracranial or base-of-skull tumours, in those with motor neurone disease and Lyme disease.

Motor Neurone Disease

This is a degenerative condition. It eventually leads to death through ventilation failure as a result of paralysis of the respiratory muscles. Different forms of the condition are seen clinically, but the one of most importance to the dental clinician is the progressive bulbar variant. In this the 'bulbar' (cranial) nerves are predominantly affected with loss of the cranial nerve motor function over a period of three to five years. This results in muscle atrophy, weakness and fasciculation of the facial and oral muscles. The eye and orbital muscles are usually spared. The most noteworthy oral aspect is the gradual inability of the patient to swallow. This will start with difficulty in managing solid foods, followed by liquids and finally problems in swallowing saliva. This can lead to drooling from the mouth and, importantly, accidental aspiration and requires direct-to-stomach feeding. Eventually the protective reflexes of the pharynx are lost and the patient dies from an aspiration pneumonia before the respiratory failure produces death. The patient often presents to a dentist complaining of excess salivation. There may be some true hypersalivation in this condition, but most of the problem results from an inability to swallow normal volumes of saliva. This can be very distressing for both the patient and the carer. The use of anti-muscarinic drugs such as hyoscine can be helpful in drying salivary secretions.

Facial Nerve Palsy (Fig 10-1)

Unilateral facial nerve palsy is the most common facial motor deficit. When there is no history or evidence of facial trauma or skull fracture this now seems related to herpes virus inflammation of the nerve and consequent loss of nerve function. The link is most obvious in Ramsay-Hunt syndrome, where there is the typical zoster vesiculation of the skin in the auditory canal and ear supplied by the sensory component of the facial nerve. The facial nerve can be affected by viral inflammation at any point in its intracranial and extracranial course, and the symptoms and signs vary accordingly. Where the forehead muscles are spared the condition is usually an upper motor lesion inside the brain such as a stroke, HIV, sarcoidosis or Lyme disease. The forehead is spared as a result of bilateral innervation to the lower motor neurone nucleus in the Pons. The classical 'Bells palsy' is a lower motor neurone lesion involving the nerve during its course through the stylomastoid canal. Consequently the only presenting feature is a unilateral facial paralysis, which can be complete or incomplete. However, lesions in other parts of the nerve can produce additional signs and symptoms, including hyperacusis, taste, lacrimal and secretory problems (Table 10-3). Management of facial nerve palsy starts with protection of the eye from corneal desiccation. This can be achieved by taping the eye shut or tarsorrhaphy (suturing the eyelids together temporarily). When CNS disease and trauma can be excluded, management of the facial palsy consists of a combination of antiviral and corticosteroid therapy. This starts as early as possible after the onset of the paralysis to reduce the possibility of a residual facial weakness, using the 'zoster' antiviral pro-

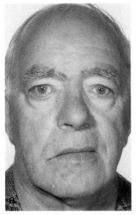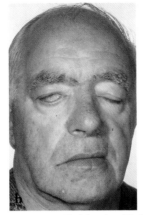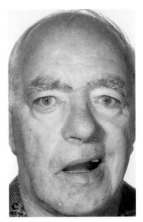

Fig 10-1 Right lower motor neurone facial palsy (Bell's palsy); (a) at rest (b) closing the eyes, and (c) smiling.

tocol. There is no equivocal evidence that high-dose steroids are beneficial, and so this treatment remains at the discretion of the clinician. Where systemic corticosteroids are used, however, this must only be in combination with an antiviral drug and at a level equivalent to 30mg prednisolone daily for one week.

If an incomplete palsy remains after one week, about 85% of patients will get full return of function, whereas only 50% with a complete palsy can expect the same outcome. Other factors that make a full recovery less likely include an advanced age of the patient at presentation, co-existing disease such as diabetes mellitus or hypertension, and the presence of additional facial nerve problems, such as hyperacusis, taste and lacrimation disturbance. Residual weakness can give a cosmetic problem as well as difficulties in oral function from loss of buccinator action. Long-term management of persistent facial weakness can be difficult, involving prosthetic enhancement or nerve-grafting in some patients.

Conclusions

- Loss of sensation or motor function is a serious symptom and demands urgent assessment and management.
- Degenerative conditions can result in significant difficulties to the delivery of dental care.

Table 10-3 **Facial Nerve Motor Loss**

Facial nerve functions
  MOTOR to second arch muscles – facial, stapedius muscle
  SECRETOMOTOR to lacrimal , submandibular and sublingual glands
  SPECIAL SENSATION taste - via chorda tympani nerve to tongue. Cell
    bodies in the geniculate ganglion
  SENSORY to part of the external auditory canal and ear

Symptoms associated with facial nerve palsy

Symptom	Lower motor neurone lesion location					Upper motor neurone lesion
	Extra-cranial	Stylo-mastoid canal	Geniculate ganglion	Intracranial course	Pontine nucleus	
Brow muscles involved	YES	YES	YES	YES	YES	NO
Facial motor loss	YES	YES	YES	YES	YES	YES
VII sensory loss	NO	NO	YES	YES	YES	NO
Hyper-acusis	NO	NO	YES	YES	YES	YES
Taste disturbance	NO	NO	YES	YES	YES	NO
Reduced salivation and lacrimation	NO	NO	NO	YES	YES	NO

Further Reading

Memory Physiology
Robertson LT. Memory and the brain. J Dent Educ 2002;66:1,30-42.

Facial Motor Loss
Gilbert SC. Bell's palsy and herpes viruses. Herpes 2002;9:3,70-73.

Salinas RA, Alvarez G, Alvarez MI, Ferreira J. Corticosteroids for Bell's palsy (idiopathic facial paralysis). Cochrane Database Syst Rev 2002;1.

Sipe J, Dunn L. Aciclovir for Bell's palsy (idiopathic facial paralysis). Cochrane Database Syst Rev 2001;4.

Oral Aspects of Neurological Disease
Fiske J, Boyle C. Epilepsy and oral care. Dent Update 2002;29:4,180-187.

Fiske J, Griffiths J, Thompson S. Multiple sclerosis and oral care. Dent Update 2002;29:6,273-283.

Alexander RE, Gage TW. Parkinson's disease: an update for dentists. Gen Dent 2000;48:5,572-580.

Mackert JR Jr, Berglund A. Mercury exposure from dental amalgam fillings: absorbed dose and the potential for adverse health effects. Crit Rev Oral Biol Med 1997; 8:4,410-436.

Chapter 11

Complementary Therapies in Oral Medicine

Aim

The aim of this chapter is to describe complementary therapies that may be used in oral medicine.

Outcome

After reading this chapter you should have an understanding of the range and value of the various complementary therapies possibly of use in oral medicine.

Introduction

Western medicine has made significant advances, particularly over the past 60 years, into the treatment of many disorders. However, these tend to only constitute around 20% of all disease, leaving some 80% at best being controlled. This applies particularly to those conditions that are chronic or have an emotional basis. In addition, modern medicine has tended to place emphasis on treatment of disease rather than its prevention including lifestyle issues. This apparent failure has resulted in a growing interest among both the general public and some health care professionals to look to alternative or complementary forms of therapy. Reasons frequently given include:
- orthodox treatments have failed
- concern over side-effects of drugs
- religious, cultural or philosophical reasons
- some people just like to protest against orthodoxy
- experiment with often exotic forms of therapy.

The difficulty for many conventional western-trained practitioners is that the mechanisms suggested as to how these therapies work do not always fit with accepted concepts of pathophysiology. In some instances reasons can be found as to why some methods such as acupuncture or hypnotherapy may be effective. In addition, the gold standard of evidence-based medicine - the double-blind randomised controlled trial - is difficult to undertake with many complementary therapies, given the individualistic nature of the treatment, such as in homoeopathy. These apparent deficits have led to a virtual rejection by many orthodox practitioners. Despite this, there are increasing numbers of patients seeking such treatment and in practitioners willing to provide it. There is also a trend in many orthodox circles towards being more open-minded and to facilitate research to determine what role these therapies may play. In addition, many medical schools, and to a lesser extent dental schools, are starting to incorporate courses covering complementary therapies within their curricula. Indeed, some therapies, such as hypnotherapy and acupuncture, are becoming accepted as routine therapeutic measures for certain conditions.

On the whole, dentistry has been slow to investigate the role of complementary medicine, with the exception of hypnotherapy. Some of the more popular therapies are discussed in this chapter. It is not all-inclusive, and interested readers are referred to the literature for more detail of the individual therapies. Those keen to pursue them further with a view to practice are recommended to seek out courses run through the various professional organisations, which are regulated, have proper codes of practice and training facilities. It is also essential to check with the medical defence organisations that they would be prepared to indemnify such therapies.

Acupuncture

Acupuncture involves the insertion of fine needles into or pressing on (acupressure) defined points within the subcutaneous tissues. It has been practiced in China for at least 3000-4000 years and probably arose from careful observation that when areas of the body were traumatised symptoms at distant points were relieved. As such, acupuncture became an important component of traditional Chinese medicine with concepts such as the five elements, Yin and Yang, the circulation of a life force Qi through meridians or channels around the body taking a well-described course. These hypotheses are difficult to understand in terms of modern science, as there is little or no evidence to support their existence. Despite this, there is clear evidence as to the effectiveness of acupuncture for a whole range of disease processes. More recent work on acupuncture has given some indication as to its mechanisms of action. These include a segmental effect, blocking the spinal gate and thereby inhibiting pain modulation. In addition, there are more generalised central effects through the raphe magnus nucleus, which is the main producer of serotonin in the brain. This may explain the beneficial effect of acupuncture on stress and anxiety. There is also an increased release of endorphins, which again could have an effect on pain perception. Acupuncture has also been demonstrated to deactivate trigger points. These are small, well-defined areas located within muscles that can become activated through stress or strain to the muscle, giving rise to chronic pain often referred to an anatomically unrelated area. Matching these trigger points, which are relatively consistent between individuals, there is a remarkable similarity to the position of a significant percentage of traditional acupuncture points.

There have been some limited trials on acupuncture in a variety of dentofacial conditions, showing beneficial effects. These include temporomandibular dysfunction, chronic facial pain and Sjögren's syndrome. There has also been a positive effect shown in helping patients control retching during intra-oral procedures, including impression-taking.

Herbalism

Herbal medicine in its various forms is probably the most ancient and indigenous form of therapy throughout the world. The use of plants, and to a lesser extent animal and mineral substances, has been passed down through folklore to treat a full range of disease. Many of these natural substances have been examined scientifically and the effective component identified. Purified forms are often produced by the pharmaceutical industry as conventional medicines. Purists argue that, by taking the active ingredients in conjunction with other components in the natural source, various toxic effects can be diminished and consequently the substance is more effective. The difficulty with using whole plants is that it is not possible to control the dosage of the active ingredient. Despite the popularity of herbal medicine there have been some disturbing reports of toxicity. There is a misconception that because plants are natural they must be safe. The popularity of herbal medicine has raised other difficulties in that there could well be interactions with prescribed medication. Practitioners need to be aware that patients may be self-administering herbal remedies, not appreciating potential dangers.

There have been some reports in the literature as to the value of certain plant preparations in oral conditions, such as recurrent oral ulceration. Most of the evidence is, however, anecdotal. As more plants are being investigated, their use in oral medical conditions remains hopeful.

Homoeopathy

Homoeopathy developed in the early 19th century with the work of Dr Samuel Hahnemann who became interested in how some plant substances, when taken, could mimic symptoms of various clinical diseases. What was more surprising was his discovery that, when taken in extremely dilute doses, these substances appeared to either ameliorate or cure symptoms of the actual disease. In practice, this is done by matching disease symptoms with those of the remedy giving rise to the basic homoeopathic principle – let like be cured by like. The principle was further extended after the observation that the effects were more pronounced the more the substance was diluted. This is done by taking the original mixture and repeatedly diluting it ten-fold with water while vigorously shaking the solution (succussed), a process known as potentisation. This last feature probably poses the greatest difficulty for the more orthodox scientific community in that in the most potent dilutions – that is to say, the most powerful - the original substance would have been diminished to the point where there are no remaining molecules present.

In addition to matching patients' symptoms with the remedy a homoeopath may also take into account a patient's constitutional make-up. This includes the possibility that a person may have been left with a chronic effect of an underlying disease that had been present in previous generations (miasms). Despite scientific doubts as to how it works, homoeopathy has remained an increasingly popular form of treatment. Remedies are readily available to the public and, unlike many conventional drugs, they are free of untoward side-effects. There have been some limited trials indicating that beneficial effects do exist for oral disease, but most are anecdotal. Theoretically, any disease that is reversible can be treated homoeopathically.

Hypnotherapy

Hypnosis has been known in various guises throughout the history of man, but its relationship with medicine has not always been harmonious. Its value in medicine progressively developed during the 19th century with its use as an analgesic and even anaesthetic agent. It was also used as a means of psychotherapy, allowing behaviour modification and symptom control. Despite these obvious benefits, hypnotherapy has remained somewhat misunderstood, surrounded by myth and extensive misuse in the name of entertainment. In spite of its somewhat shady past, hypnosis has emerged as an extremely useful tool in various medical disciplines. It is one of the few therapies to have made a significant inroad into dentistry with its use in relaxation, anxiety/phobia control and pain modulation. Any condition that has a significant emotional component could theoretically benefit from hypnosis. Great care has to be taken, however, when treating patients in relation to the suggestions given. The technique is generally considered unsuitable for patients with a history of psychosis and, unless undertaken by a specially trained practitioner, depressive illness.

There has been endless debate as to how hypnosis works. It is almost certainly a natural state akin to daydreaming, losing oneself in a book or film, with a concentrated mind that has become disengaged from other external stimuli. The hypnotist in essence acts as a teacher, instructing patients how to go into a trance state. Once there, suggestions relating to pain control, anxiety relief or even habits such as smoking are made. Relating directly to the subconscious mind allows a passive acceptance by the recipient without analysis from the conscious parts of their brain. Anyone who wants to be hypnotised can be, providing they have the ability to concentrate, although the depth of trance can vary. Children make particularly good subjects, as they have more active imaginations. There is increasing evidence as to the effectiveness of hypnotherapy. Many now regard it as a versatile adjunct to clinical care.

Osteopathy/Chiropractic

These two forms of complementary therapy involve manipulation of the joints. Although developed separately, they have many facets in common, but chiropractic has traditionally concentrated more on the spinal column and nervous system. As a result both systems are frequently used in the treatment of musculoskeletal problems. In addition they have a role in managing internal dysfunction that may have arisen due to postural problems or compression of spinal nerves. There is increasing evidence to support many of the concepts of both osteopathy and chiropractic. Both professions have regulated themselves to the point of being accepted into the realm of mainstream health care.

Groups arising out of these techniques, such as cranio-sacral osteopathy, have developed and are advocated in the management of facial pain and headaches, including temporomandibular dysfunction. Aspects of this type of treatment are frequently promoted with theoretical physiological explanations, including movement of the cranial bones and alterations in the flow of cerebrospinal fluid. These techniques may form a useful adjunct to dental therapy, in particular, with temporomandibular dysfunction.

Amalgam

It would not be possible to discuss complementary therapy without mentioning the controversy over the continuing use of dental amalgam. Slow mercury release from amalgam restorations has been blamed on a whole variety of general health problems, including chronic fatigue, multiple sclerosis, functional bowel problems and various dermatological disorders. The list is almost endless. The problem for the dental profession is that amalgam is an extremely versatile and useful material, which has been around for approximately 150 years. As a consequence its properties are well understood. In addition, despite being blamed for numerous health problems, there is a lack of tangible evidence for its toxicity. There is also some concern that chemicals released from alternatives such as composite restorations could be targets for similar health concern. Generally, the times when mercury levels from amalgam restorations are likely to be highest are during its insertion and removal. In any patient who is sensitive to amalgam (for instance, lichenoid reaction) removal should be undertaken under rubber dam isolation.

Many patients with chronic ill health who seek a solution through an alternative medical practitioner are often subjected to 'tests' to try and identify likely cause(s) of their symptoms. These tests frequently involve 'energy' measurements taken either directly from the patient through 'acupuncture points' or from samples such as hair or nail clippings. Although these tests often produce what looks like highly scientific data, very few have been evaluated and as such their significance is questionable. A number of patients seeking such investigation may be informed that dental amalgam is the cause of their problems and are advised to have their restorations removed. In some cases, other causes for their symptoms may be found, such as food intolerance or emotional issues, but in those who persist in their concern over amalgam, measurement of blood and urine mercury levels can be undertaken. This whole area is extremely controversial. Until more evidence is forthcoming, it would be difficult to recommend having restorations removed for non-dental reasons.

Other Treatments

The therapies discussed form a small fraction of those available. These range from various touch/massage therapies, dietary regimens, exercise therapies through to more contemplative relaxation techniques. Although all these methods have their advocates, evidence as to their effectiveness is often lacking, but many of the concepts should not be dismissed without appropriate research.

Conclusions

- A number of complementary therapies are available.
- The evidence base for many is lacking.
- Further research into complementary methods is needed.

Further reading

Zollman C, Vickers A. ABC of Complementary Medicine. London: BMJ Books, 2000.

Varley P. Complementary Therapies in Dental Practice. Oxford: Wright, 1998.

Appendix A

History, Examination, Investigations and Treatment Protocols

This section of the book reviews features of the history or treatment-planning for six common oral medicine conditions. These suggested protocols should be used in conjunction with the general history and examination guidelines given in Chapter 1. Each of the protocols gives focus to the more detailed history or examination needed when considering each diagnosis.

1. Lichen Planus

The following points within the complete history and examination are particularly important when suspecting a diagnosis of lichen planus.

History
- What is the complaint – roughness of the mucosa, pain, blisters or ulcers?
- Duration, periodicity and intensity of symptoms
- Extra-oral symptoms – itchy skin lesions on the arms, legs or trunk
- Precipitating and relieving factors
- Medication history from six months before symptoms began
- Treatments tried and effect of these remedies

Examination
- Oral mucosal surfaces involved
  – buccal (left and right), gingivae, tongue, floor of mouth (FOM), lips
- Skin sites involved
- Clinical type – reticular, atrophic, erosive, papular, bullous, desquamative gingivitis
- Relationship to restorations – amalgam, composite, other?

Investigations
- Clinical Photograph
  - Print - to allow changes to be noted at follow-up
- Blood tests (ONLY if lesion symptomatic)
  - Full blood count (FBC)
  - Urea and electrolytes (U&Es), liver function tests (LFTs), thyroid function, serum ferritin
  - Blood glucose

- Biopsy – Histopathology and immunofluorescence if gingival lesions present.

Lichen Planus (Biopsy Proven) Treatment Plan

No symptoms
- Reticular and atrophic– consider review only
- Erosive – review 6/12 intervals when stable – patient to contact earlier if problems arise

Symptomatic
- Lichenoid – consider amalgam replacement or altering drug therapy as appropriate
- Erosive and atrophic lichen
  - Change toothpaste, especially if there is desquamative gingivitis
  - Topical steroid regimen to control symptoms
  Consider systemic steroid treatment if topical unhelpful or symptoms severe

2. Recurrent Oral Ulceration

The following points within the complete history and examination are particularly important when suspecting a diagnosis of recurrent oral ulceration (ROU).

History
- What is the complaint – pain, blisters or ulcers?
- Number of ulcers in each attack
- Sites predominantly involved
- Duration of ulcers
- Duration of ulcer-free period
- Periodicity of ulcers
- Duration of pain from each ulcer
- Extra-oral symptoms – genital, ocular?
- Precipitating and relieving factors
- Gastrointestinal disease – altered bowel habit? rectal bleeding?
- Medication history since six months before symptoms began
- Treatments tried and effect of these remedies
- If the ulcers are predominantly tongue tip and lateral tongue lesions, stressful life events and awareness of nocturnal clenching

Examination
- Mucosal surfaces involved
  - buccal (left and right), upper/lower labial mucosa, tongue, floor of mouth, palate
- If the history suggests genital ulceration it may be appropriate to examine the genital tissue. This should be performed in a suitably private setting by an experienced physician
- Clinical type
  - non-aphthous type (trauma/viral)
  - aphthous type (minor, major, herpetiform)

Investigations
- Clinical Photograph
  - if a lesion is present on examination
  Print for records – this helps if there is future uncertainty about the diagnosis
- Blood tests – ALL patients
  - FBC
  - Folic acid and vitamin B_{12}
  - U&Es, LFTs, thyroid function, ferritin
  - Glucose
  - Coeliac screen – tests may vary according to local laboratory protocols. If available, a tissue transglutaminase should be performed, and if positive an antiendomyseal antibody test should be requested
- Biopsy – if the ulcer is not obviously aphthous in nature or has duration greater than three weeks
- Delayed and immediate hypersensitivity tests
  When there is a poor response to topical treatment

Recurrent Oral Ulceration Treatment Plan
Non-aphthous ulceration
- Identify any cause and eliminate
- Review until fully healed

Aphthous – deficiency state
- Ferritin low – iron replacement therapy
  - Ferrous sulphate 200mg, three daily for three months
  - review then and check ferritin level and symptoms change again
- B_{12} or folate
  - raised mean corpuscular volume (MCV) may indicate this

      – full dietary history may suggest a low dietary intake
      – refer to physician for investigation and correction
      – review three months after treatment commences

Aphthous – no deficiency state

- If only mildly symptomatic use a chlorhexidine mouthwash during periods of ulceration
- Recurrent trauma induced aphthae
  - manage trauma source (clenching) – for example, lower soft occlusal coverage splint
- Topical steroid delivery – more significant symptoms
  - commence AS SOON AS ulcer begins – most benefit at that time
  - frequency of application can be increased at early stages of ulcer
  - stop use of steroid when ulcer heals
  - review after three months

Consider systemic steroid treatment if topical unhelpful and no sensitivies are identified on allergy-testing

3. White Patches

The following points within the complete history are particularly important when suspecting a diagnosis of a white patch.

History

- Who noticed lesion?
- Symptomatic or not
- Extra-oral symptoms – skin rashes
- Precipitating and relieving factors – obvious trauma to area
- Smoking and alcohol history
- Medication history since lesion appeared (if known)
- Treatments tried and effect of these remedies

Examination

- Oral mucosal surfaces involved
  - buccal (left and right), gingivae, tongue, FOM, lips
- Skin involved – which sites
- Clinical appearance
  - size, surface characteristics, colour, homogeneous?
  - obvious causative factors

Investigations
- Clinical photograph
  Print to allow changes to be noted at follow-up
- Biopsy – Histopathology and immunofluorescence if indicated, especially for gingival lesions

Treatment Plan
- Eliminate aetiological factors (if any)
- If there is no dysplasia – consider review
- Mild or moderate dysplasia + candida - fluconazole 50mg/day for 14 days
  – review after this initially every 2/12
- Severe dysplasia/carcinoma in-situ/carcinoma
  – follow local protocol for management of potentially malignant lesions

Geographic Tongue and Median Rhomboid Glossitis (MRG)

Usually asymptomatic - ALWAYS consider another cause for patient's symptoms if a sore tongue is the predominant complaint - discomfort from a geographic tongue and MRG is a diagnosis of exclusion

If geographism or MRG is decided as the likely cause, consider the following plan:
- Biopsy of tongue lesion (not routinely done for geographic tongue)
- Photograph tongue to demonstrate lesion for the clinical records
- If mild symptoms, use chlorhexidine mouthwash 0.1-0.2% as required or benzydamine mouthwash as an alternative
- For moderate or severe symptoms try fluconazole 50mg/day for 14 days and review after one month
- For geographic tongue only try soluble zinc (solvazinc), one tablet three times daily for three months as a mouthwash - review in further three months

4. Sore Lips - Cheilitis/Angular Stomatisis

History
- Who noticed lesion?
- Duration of lesions
- Symptomatic or not
- Intra-oral symptoms – denture problems, discomfort
- Debilitating medical disease or immune suppression - local/systemic?
- Precipitating and relieving factors – obvious trauma to area

- Smoking and alcohol history
- Denture history and denture hygiene
- Social history - occupational or social sunlight exposure
- Treatments tried and effect of these remedies

Examination
Extra-oral
- Facial hands and scalp skin - sun related lesions (keratoses/basal cell lesions)
- Colour change in lips - white/red
- Crusting/cracking/ulceration of lips - upper and lower
- Angular stomatitis - dry, moist, erythema, crusting, size of skin involvement

Intra-oral
- Denture hygiene
- Mucosal erythema/candidiasis

Investigations
- Clinical photograph
  Print to allow changes to be noted at follow up
- Biopsy – histopathology (for persistent lip lesions)
- Microbiology swabs for angular stomatitis
  send in transport medium provided with the swab for fungal and bacterial samples and ask for CULTURE and SENSITIVITY, especially for candida and Staphylococcal species. Check with local laboratory how they would like the samples sent
  - Left and right angles of mouth (one swab each)
  - Palate
  - Upper denture fitting surface (smear or imprint test)
  - Both nostrils (one swab only)
- Blood tests – for all patients
  - FBC
  - U&Es, LFTs, thyroid function, ferritin
  - Glucose

Treatment Plan
Cheilitis
- Eliminate aetiological factors if any noted.
- No/mild dysplasia - advise sun block every day (even if the sun is not obvious) to reduce further damage.
  Hydrocortisone ointment (for short periods) or preferably a moisturising

agent can be used daily to reduce cracking or crusting - review six-monthly
- Moderate dysplasia - advise sun block review four-monthly
- Severe dysplasia/carcinoma in-situ
  - follow local protocol for potentially malignant lesions

Angular stomatitis
- Eliminate systemic factors - especially iron deficiency, hypothryoidism and Type 2 diabetes mellitus
- Educate and instruct in adequate denture hygiene measures – this is ESSENTIAL
- Consider use of topical therapy for advanced cases - NOT for every patient - miconazole and hydrocortisone ointment

5. Oral Dysaesthesia

The following points are particularly important when seeing a new patient suspected of having an oral dysaesthesia. Remember that this can be of ANY sensory modality
- Burning – no mucosal abnormality
- Dry mouth – saliva present in adequate quantity
- Bad taste/loss of taste – no infective cause/halitosis
- Tingling/disturbed sensation (no objective sensory loss)
  - no cranial nerve or local abnormality

History
- Duration and periodicity of symptoms
- Intensity of symptoms – pain scores
- Extra - facial symptoms – dyspepsia, irritable bowel syndrome (IBS), neck and shoulder pain, back pain
- Precipitating and relieving factors
- Medication history – changes over course of the symptoms
- Treatments tried and effect of these remedies
- Sleep pattern
- Social history (employment issues, family issues)

Examination
- Mucosal surfaces involved
  - buccal (left and right), gingivae
  - tongue - dorsum, tip, lateral margins
  - floor of mouth, lips, palate
  - throat and other

- Appearance of parafunction (tongue/buccal mucosa-ridging)
- Saliva presence – normal, reduced, minimal
- Masticatory muscles – normal, tender

Investigations
- Blood tests (all patients)
  - Zinc (only for TASTE disturbance)
  - FBC
  - Folic acid and vitamin B_{12}
  - U&Es, LFTs, thyroid function, ferritin
  - Glucose
- Hospital anxiety and depression (HAD) scores (all patients)

Treatment Plan
- Deficiency states – correct first
  - iron deficiency treated first, then zinc
  - B_{12} or folate
  - raised MCV may indicate this
  - refer to physician for correction – review in three months
  Ferritin low – iron replacement therapy
    - Ferrous sulphate 200mg, three daily for three months
    - review then and check ferritin level and symptoms
  Zinc low – zinc replacement therapy
    - Solvazinc 125mg three times daily for three months (warn about gastrointestinal upset)
    - review and check zinc level and symptoms

- No deficiency state
  - Tricyclic antidepressant or clinical psychology treatment
    e.g. dothiepin or amitriptyline
  - dose 50-75mg at night - review two months
  - remember drug interactions, glaucoma, prostatism
  - good for patients with poor sleep pattern and systemic anxiety symptoms
  - higher dose leads to quicker resolution

Warn about:
- drowsiness – worst in first week
- dry mouth
- blurred vision (rare)
- slow onset of action – four to six weeks for dysaesthesia
- treatment length four to six months

Review in two months – patient to contact if adverse reactions before then

Clinical Psychology
Refer for assessment if:
– patients not keen for drug therapy
– have plenty of time for visits and distance not a concern
– need to control systemic anxiety symptoms rather than alleviate them

Review after clinical psychology treatment or 6/12, whichever sooner

6. Temporomandibular Disorders (TMD)

The following points are particularly important when seeing a new patient suspected of having TMD. Remember that the symptoms vary considerably from person to person and the key to the diagnosis is often in the pattern of the symptoms

History
- What is the complaint – pain, clicking, locking?
- Description of pain – for example, throb, piercing, shooting, ache, burning
- Duration of symptoms
- Periodicity of symptoms
- Intensity of symptoms – pain scores /HAD scores
- Extra-facial symptoms – dyspepsia, IBS, neck and shoulder pain, back pain, fibromyalgia, myalgic encephalitis (ME)
- Precipitating and relieving factors
- Medication history
- Treatments tried and effect of these remedies
- Sleep pattern - difficulty getting to sleep, early morning waking
- Social history

Examination
- Extra-oral palpation – facial and cervical muscles for tender areas
- Palpation of TMJ whilst opening – crepitus, deviation, click
- Intraoral – dental state/dentures, mucosal condition (tongue crenation)
- Masticatory muscles - tenderness to palpation or forced movements

Investigations
NONE routinely indicated

Dental panoramic tomograph (DPT) radiograph ONLY if joint pathology suspected – for example, marked crepitus or locking

Diagnosis

- TMD patients usually have muscle pain on testing and a variable but diffuse pain centred around the TMJ/ear. Often there is evidence of clenching (tongue crenation and buccal mucosal ridging) and systemic associated disorders – for example, dyspepsia and IBS
- TMD has NO destructive joint lesions. It is UNLIKELY that TMD is the diagnosis if the predominant symptom is LOCKING of the mandible, either open or shut. These patients are most likely to have an internal joint derangement and should be considered for assessment by magnetic resonance imaging (MRI) and/or arthroscopy
- Patients with joint crepitus and pain on movement with arthritic changes of the TMJ on radiography (and usually other arthritic joints) may be helped by intra-articular steroid injections.
- Patients with clicking and a predominant complaint of NOISE rather than PAIN should be given treatment as below but should be informed that a successful outcome is less likely than in the treatment of pain.

Treatment Plan

First visit
- Cognitive behavioural therapy (CBT) – reassurance, advise strict soft diet, avoid wide opening
- Regular analgesia – for example, ibuprofen 400mg three times daily for two weeks
- Impressions for lower occlusal coverage appliance

Second visit
- Review progress and reinforce CBT
- Fit lower appliance - wear at night time only
  - give oral hygiene instructions
  - review after two months

Third visit
- Review progress
- If good improvement continue with appliance and final review after three months
  - educate to reduce appliance wear when symptoms settle
  - keep appliance for next episode – early treatment

- If no/poor benefit add tricyclic medication (for example, dothiepin 50–75mg at night) - review two months
  - remember drug interactions, glaucoma, prostatism
  - warn about:
       drowsiness – worst in first week
       dry mouth
       blurred vision (rare)
       slow onset of action – two to three weeks for TMD

Fourth visit
- Review effect of treatments to date – if no progress refer to appropriate specialist colleague.

Appendix B

Steroid Treatment Protocols

Topical Steroid Regimen
Aim – lowest dose to control symptoms with lowest frequency possible

Becotide 100 MDI (Metered Dose Inhaler)
- Two to three puffs in close contact directly ONTO lesion, three or four times daily
- DO NOT rinse out mouth after use
- Stop when symptoms are controlled
- Initial device from clinic – instruct patient in the correct use of the device
- Repeat prescription through general medical practitioner (GMP) as needed

Betnesol Mouthwash (0.5mg betamethasone sodium phosphate)
- Dissolve one to two tablets in 10ml of water
- Use as a mouth rinse for at least one minute – hold over symptomatic lesions
- Spit out rinse – do not swallow
- Use three to four times daily as dictated by severity of symptoms
- Letter to GMP requesting prescription (usually 100 tabs initially)
- Repeat prescription from GMP

Systemic Steroid Regimen
CHECK – Weight, pulse, blood pressure, CVA risk, diabetes - if satisfactory ask the patient's GMP to prescribe:

- Prednisolone (5mg tabs usually dispensed)
- 40mg daily for five days (if severe symptoms)
- 20mg daily for five days
- 10mg daily until review (two to three weeks)

When stable, gradually reduce systemic steroid dose – if necessary consider alternative immune suppressant drugs such as azathioprine

Systemic Steroid Side-Effects
- muscle-wasting

- thin, paper-like skin
- easy bruising
- osteoporosis
- poor wound-healing
- moon face
- centripetal fat
- amenorrhoea
- hirsuitism
- hyperglycaemia
- hypertension

Index

Quintessentials for General Dental Practitioners Series

in 50 volumes

Editor-in-Chief: Professor Nairn H F Wilson

General Dentistry, Editor: Nairn Wilson

Implantology in General Dental Practice	available
Cultural and Religious Issues in Clinical Practice	Spring 2006
Dilemmas of Dental Erosion	Spring 2006
Managing Orofacial Pain in Practice	Autumn 2006
Denatl Bleaching	Autumn 2006

Oral Surgery and Oral Medicine, Editor: John G Meechan

Practical Dental Local Anaesthesia	available
Practical Oral Medicine	available
Practical Conscious Sedation	available
Practical Surgical Dentistry	Spring 2006

Imaging, Editor: Keith Horner

Interpreting Dental Radiographs	available
Panoramic Radiology	Spring 2006
Twenty-first Century Dental Imaging	Autumn 2006

Periodontology, Editor: Iain L C Chapple

Understanding Periodontal Diseases: Assessment and Diagnostic Procedures in Practice	available
Decision-Making for the Periodontal Team	available
Successful Periodontal Therapy – A Non-Surgical Approach	available
Periodontal Management of Children, Adolescents and Young Adults	available
Periodontal Medicine: A Window on the Body	Spring 2006

Endodontics, Editor: John M Whitworth

Rational Root Canal Treatment in Practice	available
Managing Endodontic Failure in Practice	available
Preventing Pulpal Injury in Practice	Autumn 2006

Prosthodontics, Editor: P Finbarr Allen

Teeth for Life for Older Adults	available
Complete Dentures – from Planning to Problem Solving	available
Removable Partial Dentures	available
Fixed Prosthodontics in Dental Practice	available
Occlusion: A Theoretical and Team Approach	Autumn 2006

Operative Dentistry, Editor: Paul A Brunton

Decision-Making in Operative Dentistry	available
Aesthetic Dentistry	available
Communicating in Dental Practice	available
Indirect Restorations	Spring 2006
Choosing and Using Dental Materials	Autumn 2006

Paediatric Dentistry/Orthodontics, Editor: Marie Therese Hosey

Child Taming: How to Cope with Children in Dental Practice	available
Paediatric Cariology	available
Treatment Planning for the Developing Dentition	available
Managing Dental Trauma in Practice	available

General Dentistry and Practice Management, Editor: Raj Rattan

The Business of Dentistry	available
Risk Management	available
Quality Matters: From Clinical Care to Customer Service	Spring 2006
Practice Management for the Dental Team	Autumn 2006
Dental Practice Design	Autumn 2006
Handling Complaint in Dental Practice	Autumn 2006

Dental Team, Editor: Mabel Slater

Team Players in Dentistry	Spring 2006
Working with Dental Companies	Spring 2006
Getting it Right: Legal and Ethical Requirements for the Dental Team	Autumn 2006
Bridging the Communication Gap	Autumn 2006
Clinical Governance	Autumn 2006

Quintessence Publishing Co. Ltd., London